OPTI-STRETCH
VERSUS
Recurrent Back Pain

EDWIN J. NEIL, M.D., M.S.

CLASSIC DAY
PUBLISHING

Seattle, Washington
Portland, Oregon
Denver, Colorado
Vancouver, B.C.
Scottsdale, Arizona
Minneapolis, Minnesota

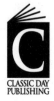

CLASSIC DAY
PUBLISHING

Classic Day Publishing
Houseboat #4
2207 Fairview Avenue East
Seattle, Washington 98102
877-728-8837
ewolfpub@aol.com

ACKNOWLEDGMENTS

■ ■ ■

This book is dedicated to my daughter Angela. She gave me the inspiration and determination to push beyond the boundaries of medicine that I had been taught. This allowed me to pursue new and exciting levels of information.

Without the help of my family members, Jack Neil, Paula Neil, Jay Neil, Terry Murray and Jerry Smith, this book could not have been written. They provided encouragement, sustenance, financial support and editing contributions. Their large families were essential in order to analyze various range of motion techniques, family tendencies and types of normal variations. They were also gracious enough to pose for some of the photographs.

A special thanks to the thousands of patients who contributed their time in allowing me to ask extensive questions about their back pain experience. Without this type of first-hand information, many of the original theories could not have been derived. Those individuals who were in the 20% that never had experienced back pain provided invaluable insight and ideas as to optimum range of motion parameters. I am indebted to the large number of patients, friends, and relatives who were kind enough to try some of the stretching exercises and submit to this type of physical examination. Of special thanks to Blake Sampson, Jayson Neil, Dayna, Sasha, JeNeil, RaeLyn, Russell, Jamie, Codie, Candace, Logan and Dakota.

Next I would like to thank the multitude of superb instructors starting from first grade throughout my 28 years of formal education. I would like to extend a special thanks to the instructors who helped teach me the skills and techniques of formal research.

I would also like to thank Dr. William Brydon, Dr. Kevin Oyama, Jayson Neil, Paula Neil, and Terry Murray for their review and helpful ideas.

While there were many unfortunate and significant set backs, I would like to thank both family and friends for their kindness and encouragement. Unfortunately, Opti-stretch may not have all the answers, but hopefully, formal scientific study will prove or disprove these new theories with larger populations. Significant breakthroughs in the relief of recurrent back pain are on the horizon for millions of individuals who battle against this problem.

While Opti-stretch may not work for everyone, I am thoroughly convinced there are literally millions of individuals worldwide that can be helped with the information found in this book. I originally went into medicine to help people. It is my sincere hope that the information in this book will be as helpful to you as it has been and continues to be for me.

TABLE OF CONTENTS

■ ■ ■

List of Exercises

LIST OF FIGURES AND TABLES

EXECUTIVE SUMMARY

■ ■ ■

Back pain negatively effects millions of individuals, alters activity levels and causes economic hardships for many Western nations.

Once the back has been severely strained, there appears to be no modality that can shorten the one to two months that are normally required to heal the injury.

Once significantly strained, several back muscles are extremely sensitive to recurrent strain patterns. Recurrent back strain syndrome is a spectrum of recurrent injury with classic signs and symptoms. In the most severe form, it can, over decades, lead to significant physical incapacity and a serious type of frequently recurring back pain.

Muscle strain has long been known as the primary cause of back pain. Yet, the precise muscle or muscles, which have been strained, still remains a question of significant controversy. Indeed, the precise cause of back pain, due to muscle strain, has long been considered an enigma. Most sufferers are told the muscle strain will eventually go away. However, after one severe strain, many individuals state that, "their back was never quite the same".

This strained area of the back then becomes extremely susceptible to reinjury. In over 2000 individuals questioned, approximately 10-25% maintained an active lifestyle and simply lived with the recurrent bouts of back strain. Later in life, due to decreased healing capabilities of the body, often the length of time necessary to heal recurrent strains would become significantly prolonged. This led to an intolerably frequent amount of strains and subsequent decrease in activity levels.

Some 50% of common back strain sufferers would continue to decrease their activity level and thereby avoid strains for long periods.

Another 25% were lucky enough to markedly rehabilitate their back. A great deal was learned from both this group, and the 20% of the total population who reported never straining a muscle in their back, despite very active lifestyles.

Opti-stretch, following extensive scientific research, has demonstrated the existence of risk factors responsible for recurrent strain to the same area of the back. If these risk factors are decreased or completely eliminated, the chance of strain recurring in the exact same location is markedly decreased. This area of the back can become optimally healed, and is no longer a "weak link".

The key, to building healthy muscles in the back, is first to tone the muscles. Later, the muscles must be strengthened and then conditioned. Without first toning the muscles, following a severe strain injury, it is difficult to strengthen the muscles, beyond a certain level. When exceeding this certain level of strength, strains will frequently reoccur. The knowledge of which muscles (i.e., psoas muscle complex) are most commonly strained in the back, allows Opti-stretch to specifically target these muscles. Once these muscles are toned, they can be rehabilitated to a healthy level.

It has long been known that there are two major functions of muscles. The first is to contract and provide movement to the body. The second function is to spasm in order to protect injuries to bones, ligaments and even the muscles themselves. This prevention of movement allows the body to heal. Opti-stretch has demonstrated that certain muscles can exist in a state of partial spasm for years and even decades. Unless, the muscles are isolated and specifically evaluated, these "asymptomatic chronically injured muscles (ACIMs)" are very difficult to detect.

Opti-stretch stretching exercises isolate the major core muscles of the back, which are responsible for the majority of recurrent back strain. ACIMs, shortened tendons and other conditions can now be identified.

Using the same stretching exercises, a process referred to as stretch receptor lengthening can often restore optimal tone to the muscles. Stretch receptor lengthening is accomplished using a specific incremental stretching technique combined with an incremental breathing technique. Over a considerable time (2 to 6 months), large increases in muscle tone can be documented.

The next important step is to strengthen the muscles. The muscles then need to be conditioned. Many good programs already exist for these two important steps.

In summary, there now exist screening tests, which can evaluate whether an individual is susceptible to recurrent back strain. Certain risk factors can be detected. This screening technique is valuable in recording the range of motion for all individuals, whether they have had back pain or not. Unfortunately, in this day and age, serious injuries from auto accidents and falls are very common. By knowing precisely where the individual's range of motion was prior to the accident, this information could be very helpful in achieving the most total rehabilitation possible.

Despite decades of recurrent back strain, many individuals have been able to significantly rehabilitate their backs. While there are several other causes of back pain, recurrent muscle strain is by far the most common. Opti-stretch has the potential for helping millions of individuals regain a healthy back.

Certain risk factors can be determined even in children. By age six, programs can be instituted to help decrease the risk factors (see Dr. Mom section). In children and young adults, the risk factors can be rapidly improved. By age 55, reduction of risk factors often becomes much more difficult. This is due primarily to age, joint injuries and arthritis.

Opti-stretch is an effective scientific program for core muscles with measurable results. It is both cost-effective and time-efficient. It is the best program I have found in my quest to leave no stone unturned in procuring a healthy back.

OPTI-STRETCH

FOR A HEALTHY BACK

■ ■ ■

CAN IT BE DONE?

CAN I DO IT?

ATTENTION TO DETAIL!

PREFACE

■ ■ ■

Bang…bang, slosh, you know perfectly well the washing machine is going to stop. The clothes have managed again…to clump on one side, and the drum bumps to a stop. Neither…mechanical machines nor the human body works well out of balance.

I have taught classes with Dr. Neil for about 2 years through the continuing education program and have seen his theories proven, over and over again with every student we've seen who complains of back pain. Those with back pain always have more limited range of motion on one side of their bodies compared to the other.

Sometimes our students bring friends to the classes for moral support. These students not complaining of back pain have equal range of motion. Sometimes they're very inflexible but still symmetrical, and the difference between the two groups of students show how tight and tender muscles can really cause debilitating pain.

The Opti-stretch screening exercises detect the weak link in the muscle and the Opti-stretch therapeutic program teaches how to return the injured muscles to an elastic healthy state.

The Opti-stretch challenge was designed to help students know what condition their muscles are in. It takes you from start to finish in rehabilitating a Chronically Injured Muscle.

The last thing you want to do is hurt the muscles when you think you're protecting them. Over-stretching can cause micro-tears and make the muscles more susceptible to injury and reinjury. It is important to understand how the intensity of stretch affects muscle health.

I have heard students say…"Thank you, thank you, you're an answer to my prayers". In our last class a student said, "I don't know why, but Opti-Stretch has really improved my belly-dancing".

The side-effects of Opti-Stretch are just about as rewarding as correcting "Asymptomatic Chronically Injured Muscles (ACIMs). Said plainly…"You just move better". The improvement in agility and posture are easily noticed. I have seen remarkable improvement in the way people move in just a few weeks.

In any sport, it's important to have the core muscles aligned and balanced, just like a washing machine. You run better and more efficiently when you're balanced and the joints suffer less stress.

Of all the exercises out there, how do you know which ones are the best? Dr. Neil has done the research and picked out 20 of the best exercises. He also had to develop a few that would best tone the core muscles of the lower back, upper back and neck muscles.

I didn't start Opti-Stretch because of a bad back. My neck was killing me from whiplashes incurred while ice-skating. Dr. Neil had me start with the back exercises, then the shoulder exercises. After that, the neck was easy to rehabilitate. It was exciting to see my movement on the ice improve, too. You'll see how differently the body works when the core muscles are symmetrical.

Enjoy…You can use this program for a lifetime. If for some reason you sustain a muscle injury, you'll know…when and how to rebalance and tone the muscles to their previous level of stretch. Opti-Stretch teaches…muscle management for a healthy back.

I still stretch the Opti-Stretch way everyday and absolutely love the program. As long as I'm stretching, why not take advantage of knowing which stretches tone the big core muscles. Even though I'm 51, have 8 kids, and overweight, I still enjoy quite an active lifestyle. And I give Opti-stretch a lot of credit for that!

Now… Dr. Neil needs to develop a weight loss program that works with such dramatic results.

– Terry Murray

INTRODUCTION

■ ■ ■

Back pain is unquestionably a major problem. It is of epidemic proportions in all first world nations. Billions of dollars are spent annually. At its current rate, economists believe some nations with socialized medicine could become economically ruined. Moreover, in its more severe form, the pain and direct negative impact on individual human lives is enormous.

This book deals only with one type of back pain due specifically to <u>muscle strain</u>. This accounts for approximately 85% of all back pain. The major focus is on low back strain that has reoccurred in precisely the same place more than twice.

Theoretically, this type of back pain should be very straightforward. A muscle or muscles become strained and cause back pain. However, despite an exhaustive effort and millions of research dollars spent between 1960 to 1995, no specific muscle has been scientifically identified, which causes this type of back pain. Even in the 21st century, the precise cause of "Benign Back Pain" is referred to in the scientific literature as "enigmatic" (something hard to understand). During the 1990's, lack of research dollars has stopped virtually all new research on back strain, except in Europe.

The only known solution is stretching or exercise programs. Physical Therapy programs are the standard for the medical profession. During the exhaustive effort to research the problem, even Yoga was formally investigated. It was determined that it offered no additional significant benefit beyond that of Physical Therapy. Due to a large public outcry that Yoga did indeed work, it was again evaluated by the medical profession with the same conclusion. Since that time, literally hundreds of various stretching programs have been published. Most are well meaning individuals who honestly believe that they have found either a specific stretch or program that can help sufferers.

So with all of the new and exciting scientific breakthroughs, what is the solution? Unfortunately, it is another stretching program. Believe me, I wished it had been a simple pill that we could take.

The stretching exercises in this program do resemble those of other programs. However, the application is significantly different. By knowing precisely which muscle is injured, other muscles indirectly effected by this injury can be determined. Complex muscle adaptation patterns occur in the human spine that protect an acutely injured muscle and allow essential movements for the body. These muscles are far larger and more powerful, thus allowing subtle adaptations that have been difficult to clinically recognize in the past. Unless these accessory and antagonist muscles are targeted and rehabilitated, the primary injured muscle cannot be fully stretched in order to become completely rehabilitated. Therefore, the muscle heals to a suboptimal level. This muscle can remain in a pain free, asymptomatic, chronically injured state for decades. The muscle tightness and asymmetry goes completely unrecognized. In this state, the muscle is far more susceptible to reinjury. Thus, a vicious cycle of recurrent muscle strain is created. No other muscles of the human body or in the entire animal kingdom, for that matter, are like this. Therefore, medicine does not believe recurrent injury cycles exist (even though everyone with a bad back would disagree). The term "recurrent back pain" was coined to identify this syndrome. This knowledge helps to explain why some individuals have done amazingly well with certain stretching programs, while others have seen little benefit.

The problem is made even more complex because it is not one muscle. Three separate muscles form the psoas muscle complex (pronounced sō´as). Well documented anatomical variations in this muscle complex account for why some individuals never have any back pain. It also explains why some can rehabilitate a strained back after a few injuries, others keep reinjuring the same muscle and why others fall into a cycle of frequent reinjury (bad back), which can be both frustrating and incapacitating.

The major breakthrough is that even after several decades and thousands of reinjuries, the psoas muscle complex can be rehabilitated. This happened to me. I was able to resume virtually any physical activity. My back has become healthy and strain resistant going on 6 years now, despite 23 years of recurrent back pain and 7 full years of very frequent reoccurrences. Others completing the program have had similar success.

The second major breakthrough is the use of stretching exercises as a screening test. Certain patterns of muscle tightness can suggest a problem. Unless corrected, there is a higher risk that acute back strain can reoccur. Certain risk factors can even be recognized in childhood and corrected (see the chapter on Dr. Mom).

This knowledge base led to other important discoveries. Muscle tone, an important but rather nebulous concept, can now be measured scientifically. This allowed the identification of a large group of individuals, who genetically have excess muscle tone. It has long been known that many hyperflexible individuals have as much or even more back pain than the general population. Recognition and improved theories as to how this can occur are presented.

The Opti-stretch program is both very specific and goal oriented. Individuals with a "bad back" can **finally see their problem**. Asymmetry risk factors can be measured and recorded. Over time, measured progress can be documented. If stretch receptor lengthening is not gradually occurring, either the program is not being correctly performed, or other anatomical factors exist. There is a completion point where the individual moves on to strengthening and conditioning the muscles, so they are optimally healthy. There also is a maintenance program.

Risk factor evaluation, therapeutic correction and life-long maintenance are the three steps of the Opti-stretch Challenge. Hundreds have been pleased with their results. Even one to two inches of stretch receptor lengthening have allowed significant increases in back health and activity levels.

Fortunately for me, the maintenance program does not require daily stretching exercises for the rest of my life, if I don't want to. By understanding alternative ways of warming up the muscles and using favorite activities to maintain muscle health, the maintenance program is used on a periodic basis to assess muscle health. With more and varied activities, the stretching exercises are needed less frequently, usually at least once a week. In this way, Opti-stretch becomes a six month rehabilitation program so stretching on a daily basis is an option and not a life-long requirement.

The knowledge gained during the program allows recognition of minor injuries in muscles and a good approach on how to rehabilitate them. This can be a valuable first aid tool for maintaining muscle health, especially as one ages.

Due to my background in comparative vertebrate anatomy and medical training in several fields dealing with back pain, the second half of the book presents more scientifically the reasons why the program works. The Appendix has very important information and work-sheets that need to be looked at (except for section B). This scientific knowledge has finally put a dent in the complex battle of "recurrent back pain", which has negatively plagued and perplexed man since earliest recorded history.

The Opti-stretch program has been presented to nearly 50 physicians, two major medical societies and two major medical universities. To date, no-one has been able to demonstrate any flaws in the logic of the anatomy and physiology presented. Many have even become very excited, but realize that it would take over $3 million just to repeat this work for medical publication. Unfortunately, in the USA, research funds for this medical problem are currently no longer available.

So, after 6 years of testing the long-term effects of the stretching exercises and techniques implemented, the program appears to be both _effective_ and _safe_ (as-long-as all of the recommendations are carefully followed). I sincerely hope it will prove as helpful to you as it has been for others and myself.

OPTI-STRETCH:
a program for optimum stretching to achieve:

1. Screening for risk factors which can lead to recurrent muscle strain (i.e., asymmetry).
2. Stretch receptor lengthening through a very narrow range, requiring attention to detail.
3. Regaining body symmetry.
4. Healing of asymptomatic chronically injured muscles (ACIMs).
5. Providing healthy strain-resistant muscles.
6. Maintenance program, which helps keep muscles healthy for life.

NOTES

_____

_____

_____

_____

_____

_____

_____

_____

_____

_____

HOW OPTI-STRETCH EVOLVED

■ ■ ■

I personally enjoy reading about the history of different authors and how various new scientific theories have evolved.

In 1997, at the age of 45, I was losing the battle with "recurrent back pain" in my own active lifestyle. My first <u>severe</u> back strain occurred at age 22 while working as a physical therapy aide. In attempting to catch a 250-pound patient from falling, I sustained a <u>severe</u> low back strain. X-ray evaluation was normal and the official medical diagnosis was "low back strain". Despite aggressive physical therapy by my employers and periodic evaluation by an Orthopedic Surgeon, the injury took almost 2 months to become pain free. I was told that it would eventually get completely better on its own. Despite returning to normal activity, my back **never quite felt the same** (until 23 years later). Multiple mild and moderate episodes of low back strain reoccurred over the next 9 years. The pain was always in the exact same location. It was always brought on by heavy lifting or twisting. The pain was easily recognizable on the right side of my low back just below the belt line over the sacroiliac joint. These recurrent strains usually healed in a few days or in just a couple of weeks. Compared to the first episode and far enough apart in months or years, they were never really considered too significant. After a couple weeks of exercise and working out, I would usually return to what I felt was full activity.

At age 31, I was very active with skiing and tennis. A senior surgery resident informed me that I was limping. I had played 6 sets of tennis the evening before and felt fine. After weeks of insistence he made arrangements for me at one of the premier Orthopedic Surgery Sports Medicine Clinics in the Northwest. I was diagnosed with a short right leg. The right leg was measured as being a full 1-inch shorter than the left. I was given the option of wearing the highest insole lift made or having my shoes built up from the bottom for a full inch. As I was having no problem at the time, I obviously elected the former. A custom-made 1/2 inch insole lift was religiously worn in the right shoe for the next 14 years.

A ski injury caused the second <u>severe</u> back strain. After four months of persistent discomfort and just not being able to get back to normal activity, I finally agreed to be seen by a friend's Chiropractor. I felt that I had benefited somewhat by the manipulation. The discomfort had definitely changed in character and it gave me hope. The exercises that were prescribed were very beneficial.

The fourth <u>severe</u> low back strain occurred at age 38. After overexerting while doing modified sit-ups on my morning work out, I felt some mild low back pain in the same old location. Hours later, I twisted slightly while reaching backwards at work. I felt the immediate onset of moderate to severe pain in my right low back area. Over the next 8 hours the pain progressed to severe pain. Due to the pain, I couldn't stand up straight. A fellow resident finally helped me stand up straight. I could barely walk due to the pain. Even lying down trying to sleep, no comfortable position could be obtained. A back brace allowed me to walk, but it was 7 days before I was able to lift anything heavier than my shoes. It would take at least 5 to 10 minutes each morning to just put on my shoes. Although, I did not have any lost time at work, there were multiple setbacks during the total 2-month healing process.

One notable problem occurred while just slightly bending forward at the waist. There was excruciating pain that caused my knees to buckle. It felt as though a knife had been stabbed in the right side of my low back. Severe pain existed in that bent knee position but trying to move either up or down was excruciating. I was simply unable to move. After being locked in that position for about 5 minutes, the pain gradually subsided somewhat and I was finally able to stand up straight again. (This is a fairly common problem with <u>severe</u> back strain.)

After 6 months I tried to ski. Having been a ski instructor, I was considered an above average advanced skier. However, I didn't progress much after starting to wear the insole lift. High performance ski boots just do not respond properly with a lift in only one boot. Even following a few gentle turns, if my low back did the slightest motion of a back bend, I would experience acute moderate back pain. The ski day was ruined. After 7 to 10 days the pain slowly resolved. During the next 4 years, I would do my routine exercises all year long to get ready for the ski season. Each year exactly the same thing would happen on the first run. Finally, after 4 annual attempts I simply gave up skiing for the next 3 years.

By age 45, I had given up skiing and snowmobiling. I couldn't comfortably pick up anything over 50 pounds even with an abdominal support binder on. I was rapidly becoming a real physical mess. I was in worse condition than some of the patients that I was treating for "chronic back pain". (**Note that "chronic back pain" is a specific medical diagnosis and has completely different reasons and pathology compared to "recurrent back pain."**)

The icing on the cake came when I could no longer lift my 3-year-old daughter over my head without back pain. She then weighed only 25 pounds. This was something she and I thoroughly enjoyed when she was little.

The above scenario is that of <u>severe</u> "benign low back strain". Only a very small percentage of the population suffers at this extreme level. However, it does account for millions of individuals in the USA alone.

I was at that time an interim director at a large University Pain Management Clinic. I formally met on a weekly basis with some of the best neurosurgeons, orthopedic surgeons, physical therapists and occupation rehabilitation specialists in the nation. The large clinical team met to discuss the chronic pain patients, the majority of who suffered from low back pain. In that capacity, I attended meetings of the American Academy of Pain Management. This particular society was unique in allowing all types of alternative medicine specialists to formally present their theories and information. With my background in research and medicine, I finally had a great opportunity to formally evaluate other alternative medicine concepts and treatments for different types of back pain. I decided that if I had to succumb to significant incapacity due to back pain and not be able to share with my daughter simple sports activities, it would only be after **leaving no stone unturned**.

At that time, I possessed a rather unique collection of knowledge including that which has already been mentioned before:

1. 17 years of practice as a MD.
2. 6 years of formal residency training including Anesthesiology and Pain Management.
3. Master's Degree in Zoology (physiology). [Note: A number of theories were generated from knowledge of animal science.]
4. 23 years of dealing with personal recurrent low back pain.

First I reviewed the medical literature again and discovered some rather obscure studies on back pain. One interesting study from England dealt with a concept of a "Short Leg Syndrome" and the relationship to back pain. I carefully reviewed all the supporting references and the reason why this theory never gained much popularity.

After one hundred years of unresolved controversy between tradition medicine and the Chiropractic community, I felt the Chiropractic field was the most likely to yield some insight into back pain. I had a fair amount of personal experience with various chiropractors. Even though I hadn't received spectacular results from chiropractors, I felt there must be a reason why I hadn't and other very reliable individuals had. Over two hundred hours were spent in the Chiropractic library, attending lectures and speaking with Chiropractic professors. Formal scientific studies were just then being jointly reported by both the Chiropractic community and the Traditional Medical community which showed no significant difference in the 1-2 month healing rate of severe back strain no matter whether Chiropractic, Physical Therapy or no therapy at all was performed.

In short, I investigated most forms of spinal manipulation including Osteopathy, Naturopathy and Feldenkrais. Each were different but each had one common theme. Movement of the body (usually through manipulation) and the return of movement seemed to be the common denominator in all the above disciplines. From my Physical Therapy background this led me to other forms of active movement therapy programs such as Yoga, Alexander technique, Callenetics, the Egoscue method and Pilates method. Various other stretching techniques were studied, including Bob Anderson, Bill Pearl, Maxine Tobias, Judy Alter and Arnold Schwarzenegger to name a few.

I evaluated over 350 stretching exercises and determined which were the safest and most effective for the specific muscles I had personally injured. Several techniques were developed to make stretching exercises more efficient (and fun). A concept of <u>stretch receptor lengthening</u> was evaluated. Martial arts and professional dance routines were evaluated. The most efficient technique to accomplish lengthening of the stretch receptors was developed.

Then, I interviewed 2000 individuals to search for similarities to my injuries. I discovered that many, many, many individuals were just like myself. They really didn't like to talk about back strain and having a "bad back". There still appears to be somewhat of a social stigma from the 70's where recurrent back pain was not felt to be real and was "all in one's head". To my dismay, this similar pathology in muscle tightness for certain muscle groups was not only common; it was <u>extremely common</u>. This condition was virtually non-existent in very young children. The incidence of this condition increased every 5 years of life to well over 60 to 80% of the individuals examined. While performing sports physical exams, I noted that the percentage of high school students with at least one asymptomatic chronically injured muscle (ACIM) detected in the upper back or neck was significantly higher than for middle school students. (Of note: due to the difficulty of examination, the low back examination was not performed.)

Gradually the theories and concepts of Opti-stretch evolved. When I presented the early discoveries to colleagues and medical societies, there was some interest but many very good questions were raised. It took several additional years of further work and research to satisfactorily answer all the questions.

After 5 years of research and testing, the evidence clearly suggests that in at least certain groups of individuals, Opti-stretch is a safe and effective form of identifying risk factors for recurrent back pain in generally <u>**healthy**</u> adolescents and adults. However, correcting these risk factors with the therapeutic techniques described in this book is not quite as safe. Unfortunately, there is a potential for injury in <u>everything</u> we do, even staying in bed all day. The Opti-stretch method, as a therapeutic program, can be potentially injurious. However, it has also safely returned hundreds of individuals to a newfound control in their lives of not being dependent on various doctors and medications when back pain would frequently <u>**reoccur**</u>. It also significantly improved their activity levels. Remember this is <u>**not**</u> a program for any back pain that is brand new to you or any acute back strain (which can often appear very similar to certain types of Chronically Injured Muscles). Nevertheless, I personally believe that Opti-stretch can and does offer a relatively safe, scientific program for improving back health which literally millions of individuals can potentially benefit from. It is the first new scientific discovery pertaining to recurrent back pain in the last 100 years.

WHAT IS OPTI-STRETCH?

■ ■ ■

Opti-stretch is an exciting new program designed to reduce or eliminate the recurrence rate of back pain in millions of individuals caused specifically by a <u>strain injury</u> to the muscles. Many stretching programs have evolved which have shown to help back strain in certain individuals. Opti-stretch optimizes the number of stretches needed, the breathing technique required and other essential techniques that changes stretching to a stretch receptor lengthening program. This allows optimal toning of muscles, which is the first step for later strengthening and conditioning muscles in order to return the muscles to a completely healthy state. Trying to strengthen poorly toned muscles is often fraught with recurrent injury to the muscles.

Unfortunately, it was not designed for all types of back pain. It is well documented that approximately 80% of the Western populations will have at least one significant episode of back pain in their lifetime. What isn't well documented, is what happens after the first significant back strain. Having interviewed thousands of individuals, there appears to be two very distinct courses of this problem. Approximately half of these individuals will, after 1-2 episodes, be able to return to their previous activity level and are considered to have regained a strong back. The other half will develop a syndrome of dozens to hundreds of recurrent back pain episodes in the exact same location. Many find that with decreasing their activity level or decreasing the weight that they lift, they are able to cope with the problem and can function in a relatively pain free state. Either consciously or subconsciously they are <u>constantly</u> aware that if certain activity levels are exceeded, the chance of re-injury to that precise area of the back is extremely high.

In youth, this is rarely a clinically significant problem because of the months or years between recurrent episodes. However, conscious or subconscious awareness of limits to their activity level can have an impact on their athletic development and choice of the activity levels that they will choose as an adult. Seldom is back strain seen much before the age of 8-12. This usually falls in the mild to moderate strain categories. The first occurrence of a <u>severe</u> strain is most frequently seen in the early 20's of an individual. Past the age of 35, this type of injury can become a serious recurrent problem. Each significant re-injury often requires an even lower activity level to avoid re-injury. Because back pain is commonly recurrent, many people are either forced to battle with it in order to gain higher activity levels or simply cope with it. By age 45-55 the recurrent injury rate can become so frequent, there are seldom any long periods of relief. In this form, it is similar to other long-term incapacitating diseases.

When I decided to "leave no stone unturned" in my search to improve my own back problems, I began by studying <u>every</u> discipline dealing with back pain. After hundreds of hours investigating the D's, (Doctors of Medicine, Chiropractic, Osteopathy and Naturopathy), I covered A to Z from Acupuncture to Yoga. At the same time I interviewed approximately 2000 people and asked them just to talk about their experience with back pain (or lack thereof). Individuals who had been diagnosed with low back strain and who had at least 2 recurrences in the exact same location were my main focus. Those individuals who described a type of victory over recurrent back pain were especially informative. It became apparent that disciplines successful in helping at least some individuals out of the vicious cycle of recurrent back pain, dealt with a concept referred to as <u>movement therapy</u>. There appeared to be at least three types of movement therapy. These types of movement therapy include self-movement by the patient (i.e., exercise, walking, or some activity), direct movement by the practitioner (i.e., Physical Therapy and Osteopathy) and indirect movement where another part of the body is moved (manipulated) to improve the injury (i.e., Chiropractic).

Strain injuries to muscles commonly result in tissue damage (bruising and microscopic damage to the muscle cells). When a muscle perceives pain either from direct injury or even indirectly from other structures in the skeletal system, the muscle goes into a <u>protective spasm state</u>. The amount of spasm is dependent on the severity of injury. This spasm protects the area from movement to allow healing. The healing process is a gradual increasing (lengthening) of pain free motion. Significantly injured muscles will continue to heal by a gradual process over days, weeks, or even months. The pain free range of motion gradually increases to a level that is functional and appears quite normal for most activities. For most individuals, when they can again do most activities without the muscle bothering them, the strain is considered healed. However, in this functional state, the muscle has often not returned to its previous level of health. In a completely healthy state the muscle must have sufficient tone, strength and conditioning. If the muscle does not completely regain the proper tone (normal range of motion) it is very difficult to properly strengthen and condition the muscle to the same level prior to injury.

This type of muscle with a chronic injury is referred to as an <u>asymptomatic chronically injured muscle (ACIM)</u>. The classic presentation of this type of injury is a previously strained muscle that for all practical purposes appears to have returned to normal. However, when the muscle is carefully assessed, it is somewhat tighter (less range of motion). The muscle will typically have $1^{1}/_{2}$ - 2 inches or more of decreased range of motion. The muscle is noticeably more tender to touch and often develops "knots" (trigger points) compared to the same muscle on the other side of the body. Also the <u>transition range</u> of stretch-to-discomfort-to-pain is noticeably different. These asymptomatic chronically injured muscles (<u>ACIMs</u>) can exist in this state for up to decades until some type of movement therapy finally returns the muscle to an improved level of muscle tone.

Every form of movement therapy that I could find was thoroughly evaluated. While researching the field of Yoga, I stumbled upon several stretching exercise programs claiming to cure back pain and prevent it from recurring. Each of these stretching programs was studied in depth. Stretching exercises have long been a tool for Physical

Therapy and a home treatment activity by the majority of medical professions. While various stretching exercises constitute a recommended treatment, there is no one set of exercises that is considered significantly better than another.

Several recent scientific studies comparing Chiropractic, Physical Therapy and no treatment at all have shown there is no currently known way to shorten healing of a <u>severe</u> back strain. Of these three types of therapy, none could shorten the 1 to 2 months that it normally takes the average severely strained back to heal. This suggests that the solution to the problem is not in shortening the healing process but preventing it from recurring again. Some type of movement therapy appeared to be the key. All the programs studied, claimed some successes in returning the injured back again to a healthy state.

Stretching and specific exercise routines had always worked for my back in the past. However, with a fourth <u>severe</u> injury to the low back and increasing age, there seemed to be a definite limit of physical activity, which I couldn't get beyond despite stretching and exercise.

To develop the Opti-stretch program over 350 different stretching exercises published in various books and magazines were then evaluated. A practical number of very specific stretching exercises were chosen that could be used daily and that isolated specific muscles of the back that were commonly prone to injury. A few new stretching exercises had to be designed. Most active individuals who had <u>never experienced any back pain</u> were able to comfortably perform the stretching exercises. However, individuals from the recurrent back pain group consistently had difficulty in comfortably performing the exercises symmetrically. New scientific theories were formulated to help explain why some stretching programs seemed to work better than others. The scientific theories also offer an explanation why some individuals achieve better results.

The stretching exercises target very specific muscles of the spine (referred to as the <u>core muscles</u>). Certain specific muscles were found to be reinjured time and time again. Sometimes the re-injury would be weeks to months apart. Commonly, these injuries could be several years apart. Stretching exercises were specifically designed to stretch and tone certain essential core muscles. One of the stretching exercises has even been used for over 2000 years. The stretching exercises are simply a tool for movement therapy. The theories, concepts and practical applications behind the stretches are what contribute to the success in the Opti-stretch program.

The major goal of Opti-stretch is to allow you personally to "run, jump, work and play with the other kids your age". It doesn't matter whether you're a kid 6 or 60 years of age. The youngest age where certain risk factors could definitely be demonstrated was at 3½ years of age. If tight, tender muscles (ACIMs) can be detected, Opti-stretch therapeutic stretching techniques have shown to lengthen the range of motion of the muscle by at least 1-2 inches in average healthy individuals. Over months, muscles have a visco-elastic property that allows the range of motion of the muscle to actually stretch further through a process referred to as <u>stretch receptor lengthening</u>. This process tones the muscle and allows for an increased level of movement and activity.

Even non-limber individuals in their 40's have been able to regain a similar level of range of motion as a <u>"3 to 5 year old child"</u>. Over 95% of all healthy 3 to 5 year olds have a very similar range of motion, referred to as the <u>"gold standard"</u> range of motion. Over this age, especially in the female population, range of motion can significantly increase. Opti-stretch has demonstrated that with the proper technique and work, even 40 year olds can develop the same level of movement that they enjoyed as a 3 to 5 year old child. If at first glance the stretches seem way too difficult, it most likely means that you are one of the individuals who could benefit most from increasing your range of motion on the tighter muscles by at least 1 to 2 inches. Keep in mind there are some individuals in their 70's who can easily perform all of the Opti-stretch stretching exercises to the level of the "gold standard". Their own activity level has maintained this level of movement throughout their life. Their activity level is in the top 10% for their given age group. They are also frequently in the 20% of the population that have <u>never had any back pain</u>.

For individuals with documented risk factors, upon completion of Step I and Step II of the Opti-stretch program, they could not only increase comfortably their range of motion but recurrent episodes of strain significantly decreased either in number or severity. For those who were able to complete the program to the level of the "gold standard" and to both strengthen and condition the muscles that had risk factors, the recurrent injury in that precise location was effectively eliminated. Consistent hard work for 20 minutes a day for 2-6 months is not easy. Using a goal oriented approach to track progress proved to be a significant motivating factor.

Unfortunately, Opti-stretch doesn't work for everyone with recurrent back strain. Individuals, with certain types of joint pain, joint injury or chronic soft tissue injury, sometimes cannot comfortably generate a sufficient amount of stretch to the muscles, without producing a sensation of pain, which results in reflex muscle spasm or injury. The muscles will then go into a protective state of partial spasm making toning of the muscle either slow or impossible. It is better to start Opti-stretch when you are age 5 rather than age 65. Opti-stretch was designed for healthy individuals without any medical conditions. Individuals over age 35 need a doctor's consent.

For those who are sufficiently healthy to participate in the Opti-stretch program, a series of specific "Challenges" are included to help in effectively and safely obtaining their goals. No one yet has obtained the "gold standard" level without significantly improving the problems with their back, if indeed the problem was due to muscle strain.

Opti-stretch is designed for only **one** of the 35 known causes of back pain. That one cause of back pain is "recurrent back strain", which is due to muscle strain. It is, by far, the most common cause of back pain.

Remember these old adages.

"To a man with a hammer,
everything looks like a nail."

"A little knowledge can be very dangerous."

"The more you know,
the more you know you don't know."

USE CAUTION:

Opti-stretch is a very powerful program! If not done properly or if tried on other stretches, it can be potentially dangerous. In testing and perfecting this program I personally incurred hundreds of minor strains to various muscles. Also (mostly from my own stupidity and aggressive nature), I incurred two separate injuries to non-core muscles which took 6 month to completely heal. Even with a developed program, I incurred a 1-week injury to core muscles of the low back testing a newly published excellent scientific technique called PNF (proprioceptive neuromuscular facilitation). Please learn the basic concepts before you try to incorporate any new variation or any stretching exercise other than those specifically described in this book.

COMMON BACK PAIN
LOCATIONS

■ ■ ■

"Common things are common."

Recurrent strains of the back, usually over time, localize to one side or the other; while many of the less serious strains are located near the midline of the back. The most common strain of the low back is felt near the midline just above the pelvis. This is usually either a mild or moderate type of strain. It usually appears due to lifting with the back instead of with the legs. The average 175-pound male can lie on his back and lift over 500 pounds with the strength of his legs. However, while standing and lifting an object with both the legs and the back in the proper squat lifting position, he can only lift 250 pounds. In a standing position with the knees kept completely straight (straight-leg dead-lift), an individual lifts only with the back muscles. This same 175-pound male can usually only lift 50-75 pounds comfortably.

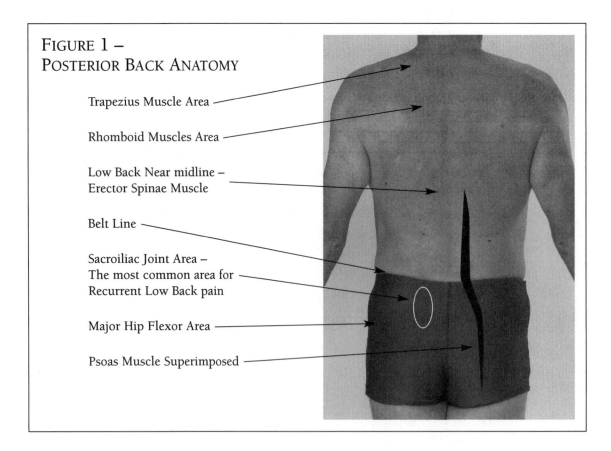

FIGURE 1 –
POSTERIOR BACK ANATOMY

Trapezius Muscle Area

Rhomboid Muscles Area

Low Back Near midline –
Erector Spinae Muscle

Belt Line

Sacroiliac Joint Area –
The most common area for
Recurrent Low Back pain

Major Hip Flexor Area

Psoas Muscle Superimposed

Most professional weight lifters will exercise and strengthen their back with the straight-leg dead-lift exercise but rarely will they push this exercise to extreme limits like the other exercises mentioned above. They are rightfully concerned about hurting

COMMON BACK PAIN LOCATIONS

their backs. Unfortunately, many health care workers, firefighters, rescue workers and blue-collar workers frequently must perform this type of suboptimal lifting in an emergency situation. Lifting with mostly the back muscles and little of the leg muscles will commonly injure this area of the low back.

Other frequent causes of midline low-back injury are repetitive bending or working in the bent-over position much of the day. Either or both of these activities will commonly lead to mild strains of the low back in the midline. This usually involves the major back muscles called the erector spinae muscles.

Another common cause of midline back pain is strain to the interspinous ligament. This condition usually involves a very specific type of injury to ligaments connected to the spine. The injury seldom takes over two weeks to heal. Rarely is there a recurrent problem, unless the same forces are again delivered to the low back.

However, "recurrent low back strain" is quite a different process, especially when strains are severe. This strain usually happens while lifting a heavy object or even lifting a light object while twisting. The pain can be immediate or it can merely feel like a moderately pulled muscle in the low back. Within 2 to 6 hours, the pain progressively becomes excruciating. During the excruciating phase of the pain, which lasts for several days, the pain is felt in a large band of the low back. Walking is barely possible and no position of comfort can be found, even while lying down. As the pain slowly eases, the individual can begin to walk with minimal discomfort. At this time, the pain generally localizes to either the left or right side over the sacroiliac area of the spine. The midline can still be tender, but is usually not the primary focal area of the pain. The most common way to make the pain worse is performing even a slight backward bending of the low back.

The severity of the pain will usually cause the individual to seek medical evaluation on the first couple of occasions. Due to the 4 to 8 weeks of pain and limited physical activity, it is usually an event that is remembered by most patients. Many individuals rank the pain on the same level as a broken bone or major surgery. The problem with this particular injury is that in various stages, it keeps reoccurring after years of being dormant. Also, the amount of force to the back, which will cause the problem to reoccur, becomes less and less with each new injury. Often, something as minor as twisting backwards to pick up a paper clip which is slightly behind them, will cause a recurrent injury that can take weeks to heal. Because the pain location is almost always in exactly the same area, the individual can usually differentiate whether the pain is simply a reoccurrence of their usual back pain, or whether it is a new and different injury.

Often, in more severe strains, there are other associated muscles and muscle groups that are also painful (i.e., accessory or antagonistic muscles). This phenomenon helps to confirm the involvement of the psoas muscle complex in this type of injury. The psoas muscle complex is one of the most complicated muscle groups in the human body. Anatomically, there is a psoas major muscle, a fusion with the iliacus muscle to form the iliopsoas muscle and a completely separate psoas minor muscle, which all form the **psoas muscle complex**. A more complete description and photos are found in the Scientific Considerations #14. The Psoas Muscle.

A muscle that is tender to the touch is an indication there is some type of injury. Tenderness of the upper psoas muscle area (see Figure 2 – Anterior Back Anatomy) can be demonstrated in a few certain body types by touching the muscle. Due to the location deep in the abdomen, the significant pressure that must be placed on the abdominal contents and the amount of adipose tissue in this area, the muscle can seldom be palpated and only in certain body types. This is a very uncomfortable area to palpate (touch) and best performed by the individual themselves.

The best way to find the area is to tighten the stomach muscles. Between the belly button and upper part of the pelvis the outside edge of the rectus abdominus muscles can be felt. Using both hands on each side of the abdomen, you slowly and gently massage deeper until touching on either side of the spine. If one side is consistently more tender this is a good indicator the psoas muscle complex on that side is involved. Remember that there is only about a 5 to 10% chance that you have the thin body type that allows this type of pressure directly on the psoas. Push slowly and carefully making sure not to press too hard.

The iliacus muscle is somewhat easier to feel. With both thumbs pressing at the same time in order to compare sides, the anterior part of iliac muscle on the inside part of the pelvic bone can be felt. In a chronic injury of the psoas complex, one side is often more tender than the other.

The upper iliopsoas muscle (another part of the psoas complex) is very easily palpated in the area of the arrow seen in (Figure 2). The fingers can easily feel the 1-1/2 inch wide muscle in this location. The large femoral nerve runs in conjunction with this muscle. Therefore, enough pressure will normally cause this muscle to feel uncomfortable. That is why both sides need to be pushed on, at the same time and in precisely the same location, in order to determine, if one side is more tender than the other.

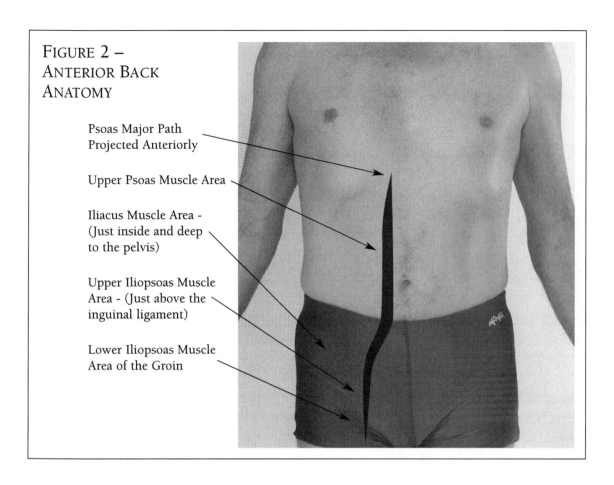

FIGURE 2 –
ANTERIOR BACK
ANATOMY

Psoas Major Path
Projected Anteriorly

Upper Psoas Muscle Area

Iliacus Muscle Area -
(Just inside and deep
to the pelvis)

Upper Iliopsoas Muscle
Area - (Just above the
inguinal ligament)

Lower Iliopsoas Muscle
Area of the Groin

The groin region is mentioned because injuries to the psoas complex after the muscle leaves the retroperitoneal space of the abdominal cavity may manifest themselves by unilateral tenderness in this area. This is referred to as a "pulled groin" and is often seen in runners.

Another rare injury in runners is abdominal pain following severe overexertion while running. Frequently they will have severe upper abdominal pain lasting days. When they return to running, the pain tends to reoccur on a mild but uncomfortable basis for weeks. The only other area of noticeable discomfort is in the groin area and is frequently treated as a pulled groin by sports trainers. It is now believed this may actually be an anterior strain injury to the upper psoas muscle. In this area the psoas muscle is outside of the upper retroperitoneal space. The associated tightness and discomfort of the iliopsoas muscle in the groin area, is due to general tightness along the entire psoas complex and is noticed where the iliopsoas leaves the lower part of the retroperitoneal space.

The lower iliopsoas muscle is felt just to the outside (lateral) of the large pulsating artery in the groin. Due to large nerves and blood vessels that are normally tender to palpation, you must compare each side at the same time and in the same place. Like the other muscles, if there is a difference you will definitely feel it. If you have a hard time deciding which side is more tender, this usually means both sides are the same. ■

The hip area is an extremely common place for lower back pain problems to manifest themselves and is more frequently seen in females. During the healing phase of a <u>severe</u> back strain, most people will remember one hip being more tender than the other to sleep on. In a few individuals, mildly injured hip muscles can become quite painful for long periods of time. It is associated with chronic injury to the psoas complex.

The hip area is frequently difficult to assess, especially in females. The easiest way is to slowly walk in place. Starting at the mid part of the thigh and along the outside edge, the bone called the femur can usually be felt. In 1 to 2 inch distances, keep feeling toward the hip. At some point, you will begin feeling muscle and the bone moving below. Feel the area 1/2 to 1 inch toward the back of this point and toward the direction of the buttocks. This is the insertion point of some of the major hip flexors of the pelvis (superior and inferior gamellus, quadratus, pyriformis, obturator externis and gluteus medius). Due to certain nerves and ligaments, this area must be felt on both sides at the same time and in the same place, to determine if there is any tenderness in this area. At times, the muscles can become so inflamed that this area can appear much like a hip bursitis.

The most common upper back injury is located between the shoulder blades and frequently involves the rhomboid muscles (see Figure 1 – Posterior Back Anatomy, page 16). Usually the symptoms are localized to only one side. A deep massage of the area or performing the Rhomboid Pull stretching exercise will frequently demonstrate that this particular muscle group is more tender on one side than the other.

Unfortunately, neck pain can be very complex and can have many different causes other than primary muscle strain. The most common location of the pain is usually along the trapezius muscle. While the mid point of the muscle is the area most commonly involved, any point along the entire muscle can manifest a chronic muscle injury state. Frequently, tenderness and knots called "trigger points" can easily be felt. The most common cause is some type of strain to the neck. The second most common cause is the neck muscle's response to lower or upper back chronic muscle injury. That is why the lower and upper back chronic injury conditions must be first healed, before any significant healing of the neck area will generally occur.

SECTION I – BASIC CONCEPTS FOR A HEALTHY BACK

■ ■ ■

Too much simplification of a complex problem can be hazardous. Remember that the primary goal of Opti-stretch is to help individuals who recurrently strain a specific part of a single muscle in the back again and again. If these individuals can rehabilitate these chronically injured back muscles, their backs will return to a normal healthy status so they can enjoy age appropriate activities, for both an active and healthy lifestyle. Whether you are a kid age 6 or 86, these concepts can help reestablish and maintain a strain-resistant back.

In sharing with you my thousands of hours of research, these concepts have the potential for helping literally millions of individuals. However, being a retired M.D., these are by no means any form of medical recommendation. In my opinion, Opti-stretch now offers an exciting and reliable program for rehabilitating the majority of "bad backs" due specifically to muscle strain. It does require a great deal of effort in simply learning the concepts and principles. Also, there is a fair amount of time commitment and work. However, the potential for helping future generations is enormous. With widespread implementation by the Dr. Mom's of the world as a basic first aid approach to recurrent back strain, their kids can enjoy virtually any active lifestyle they choose and not develop <u>recurrent back strain syndromes</u>. Remember, this doesn't mean they will not strain their backs on occasion. It means that these occasional strains will not be converted into a "recurrent back strain syndrome".

There is often a direct correlation between an active lifestyle and a healthy back. The concepts of a healthy back and active lifestyle are simple for the average person to understand. However, they are extremely difficult to specifically define and measure from a scientific standpoint. For example, if you have a bad back, what are the criteria to say you have moved from a bad back to a healthy back? Regarding active lifestyles, at which point do you move from a "normal" or average lifestyle to an above average life-style (i.e., certain Olympic athletes)? Is there a basic activity that an individual can perform comfortably which insures they have a healthy back (i.e., similar to professional movers or heavy laborers)?

A good current working definition for a healthy back is having a back that lets you enjoy any activity you want, without constantly having to worry about reinjuring the back. Being able to "run, jump, work, play and keep up" with the other kids your age not only confirms back health but also improves overall general health. Currently, only 20% of the population will reach age 45-65 without ever having experienced a single day of back pain. Of the 2000 individuals interviewed at the outset of the Opti-stretch research, some 400 individuals were found in this "never any back pain" category. This group was extremely helpful and insightful in defining from a scientific standpoint what a healthy back actually might be. For most of us with recurrent back pain, it is hard to even imagine an individual being so lucky.

Could it be that these individuals never really did much; so consequently, they never hurt their back in the first place? Just the opposite was found. Many were blue-collar workers with very strenuous jobs and others were professional athletes. All were found to have very active lifestyles simply because they never had experienced any type of back pain. This means, they never had to worry about hurting their backs. They simply did whatever they wanted! In all of my research, I had never encountered a single research article dealing with this group and what makes them so different from the other 80% of the population.

In contrast, the individuals suffering from multiple severe bouts of recurrent back pain due to simple lifting strains were just the opposite. Activity levels were generally lower in this group. Also, if they did perform higher activity levels, these levels were both carefully chosen and cautiously performed so as not to reinjure their backs.

There appeared basically three different groups based on personality types. The first group was very activity minded. They were determined not to let back pain get in the way of their life goals. They often succeeded in regaining a very active lifestyle and were able to perform strenuous work. These individuals are referred to as the "activity rehabilitation group".

Another group of individuals was also found to be equally very activity minded. They kept pushing and working to regain the active lifestyle they wanted following a significant back strain. Sometimes, the back would even be pain free for 5 years or more. Unfortunately, some activity would eventually flare up the identical back pain again. Sometimes, it would be heavy lifting or strenuous activity. However, sometimes an activity as simple as twisting to pick up a paper clip would throw the back into spasm. Many described their backs as having a "bad back" or a "trick back". No matter how hard they tried and exercised, they were able to progress only to a certain level. These individuals described their back as "never being quite the same" following their initial significant injury.

While young, these individuals considered themselves pretty normal because of the long intervals between bouts of back pain. However, by age 25-35, the recurrent injuries would become much more frequent. Also, the amount of weight lifted that would cause the reinjury, steadily decreased to such a level that they were eventually forced to start avoiding or even giving up various activities. This group was referred to as the "persistent reinjury group". I was a member of this group.

A third group was found. Each time the back pain reoccurred, these individuals would simply reduce their activity level. Eventually, the problem would go away. This is a very common phenomenon of "benign back pain" and the primary reason why after age 65 the incidence of <u>severe</u> back strain significantly decreases.

A classic example was the lady who stated she had never had back pain on a questionnaire. In reviewing her old records, I found she had several visits to the clinic for benign back strain. When asked about the back pain some 2 years prior she responded, "Oh that back pain. That all went away when I quit doing housework". This group religiously avoided certain activities. By decreasing their activity level sufficiently, the back pain would not be a significant problem and appear to have gone away. This group was called the "<u>inactivity coping group</u>". However, if this certain self-imposed activity level was exceeded and they, for some reason, returned to what would be considered normal activity for their age, reinjury frequently occurred.

Approximately 15% of all individuals with back pain reported some type of known pathology. Surgery, arthritis, a severe accident, a broken bone or a herniated disc were some of the more common pathologies responsible for this group's back problems. In this group, the only individuals who were extensively questioned and examined, were those who had essentially returned to normal activity levels.

If this small study is any indication of the general population, the "<u>persistent reinjury group</u>" may constitute approximately 20% of the general population. This would amount to approximately 20-50 million individuals in the USA alone. This group displays certain similar physical characteristics and is referred to as having a "recurrent back strain syndrome".

"Recurrent Back Strain Syndrome" can be described as back pain that classically arises from some type of lifting injury that caused significant (either moderate or severe) back pain. This condition very seldom occurs in young children. Seldom does it start before age 13. Most commonly, the first significant strain occurs in ages 20-25. Many are seen by their doctors. Having practiced for 7 years in Emergency Rooms and Urgent Care Clinics, I am very familiar with what often happens. After a history and physical examination to assure there is no neurologic injury, an x-ray is often taken. The diagnosis in the vast majority would be that of "low back strain". Although strain is often diagnosed, this examination is very important in order to make certain that no type of pathologic back pain exists.

In <u>severe</u> back strain cases, usually medications are prescribed and the individual is referred to a Physical Therapist (depending on insurance). In the mid 1990's, several good studies have shown that regardless of the treatment (including Chiropractic), the injury would heal in the same 1 to 2 months. The majority of these individuals would return to normal activity following the first severe strain. However, many reported to me the same thing that I had experienced. Even though after 2 months of healing and essentially able to return to the same activity level, "the back just never felt the same".

Over this 1 to 2 months, the back does not heal at a steady rate. Instead, the average person usually has multiple setbacks and minor reinjuries. The analogy is a badly sprained ankle. Once evaluated medically and determined to be a sprain, the ankle eventually goes on to heal. However, as the ankle gets feeling better, there would be a number of mild or moderate sprains (strains) before it would eventually heal. It is not like a broken bone (which I have also experienced several times). After the cast goes on, each day there is a little improvement until the pain is gone. There is a long pain free period until the cast comes off. The limb is weak and most extensive movement is quite painful. However, the limb rapidly returns to normal over a one or two week period. Seldom are there reinjuries or setbacks, unless a joint or severe muscle strain has occurred with the broken bone.

In sharp contrast with the broken bone, a moderate or severe back strain will usually always have several reinjuries before it completely heals. Each is usually less severe than the one before. Eventually the periods between these strains lengthens until the area eventually returns to normal. This is something that the average individual learns to expect as a normal healing pattern. Also, they quickly learn which activities will usually cause mild reinjuries or setbacks. This is one of the reasons why, following 2 or 3 similar recurrent strains in exactly the same area, the individual recognizes they just have a strained muscle. Seldom do they seek medical attention. The reinjury again heals with multiple setbacks. Sometimes "zingers" will occur. These are sharp pains in that same area, which warn the individual that they are over-doing. The sharp pain that can then shoot down the leg or up the back, lasts only seconds. Once gone, the back usually seems all right. Most continue what they are doing, but try to avoid the exact twisting or lifting activity for at least several hours.

After a couple of trips to the Emergency Room or doctor's office in which they are told that their back is simply strained and it will eventually heal, many will self-diagnose the back pain in that same location as another reinjury. Frequently, they quit seeking further traditional medical attention for this problem. Many try Chiropractic, Naturopathy or Osteopathy treatment. There were 19 million visits to chiropractors alone in 1998. Many of these individuals reported that the pain would go away sooner. However, in many cases, these same individuals would find that the back pain still kept periodically returning.

At that point, many will just quit returning to physicians and simply learn to live with the problem. Most try not to spread the fact that they have a "bad back", and prefer not to talk about it with others. Therefore, traditional medicine has poor data about the natural history of this particular disease. In medical school, the above scenario is taught as a more severe pattern of benign back pain. The major difference is that following each injury, the muscle is believed to completely heal similar to the healing process of a broken bone. It is taught that the strained muscle will heal usually stronger and there should be no reason for that particular muscle to again become strained, unless there are significant strain forces in that location so as to damage (strain) the muscle again. Also, it is taught that the disease of benign back strain is usually self-limiting by age 65. This most likely occurs due to much lower incidence of heavy lifting at that age. So the disease usually does **eventually** go away.

For those with the mild or moderate forms of "Recurrent Back Strain Syndrome", they essentially enjoy a normal life with the exception that their "trick back" will occasionally "go out". For those who have the severe form, it is entirely a different story. A full 2 months to heal the pain is very incapacitating. Put into perspective, each time these individuals severely strain their back is just like the average person breaking a bone and needing a cast applied.

Many are forced to give up certain dreams regarding the various physical activities they like to perform in life. Many find their general activity level falls significantly below normal. This can have a serious effect on their happiness and their potential accomplishments in life. Also, the trillions of dollars spent annually by these subgroups in trying to cope with this condition are significant. Even worse yet, the <u>severe</u> recurrent pain category is not recognized as the truly incapacitating disease entity, which it can be. Socially, individuals in the <u>severe</u> recurrent back strain groups are compared with the milder forms of this recurrent problem. Many report that family and friends often blame them for not being able to better cope with this problem.

The key to the scientific discoveries of Opti-stretch was in being able to talk comfortably with individuals in a non-threatening situation so they were very open about their condition. By then comparing and contrasting the "<u>never any back pain</u>" with the "<u>activity rehabilitated group</u>" and the "<u>persistent reinjury group</u>" important data was generated. This led to a review of Hippocrates' early work in 400 BC. The "father of medicine" showed the importance of "movement therapy". Much of this information was lost to the West during the Dark Ages. However, it appeared to be somewhat preserved in the East, which 800 years later became known as Yoga. Some believe that the "movement therapy" knowledge base also helped contribute to the emergence of several types of manipulation that arose in the USA during the late 1800's (i.e., Chiropractic and Osteopathy).

Traditional medicine adopted the specialty of Physical Medicine and relegated the more common forms of rehabilitation to Physical Therapists. However, for the "Recurrent Back Strain Syndrome" groups, the above mentioned treatments were often not completely successful. Healing arts and programs like American Yoga, Pilates, Callanetics, Egoscue technique and hundreds more emerged. Some reported significant successes. The prototype of "movement therapy" has been that of Yoga. It is frequently heralded as a 2000-year-old program that can help back pain. However, when twice formally evaluated by the American Medical Association, there appeared no significant benefit that would promote adoption into mainstream medicine. In my interviews, several individuals stated that they had tried Physical Therapy and had finally found relief in non-traditional movement therapy programs. It became apparent these various programs were valuable in helping at least certain types of benign back pain. However, why would one individual benefit and become significantly rehabilitated, while another would continue to suffer with recurrent injuries?

Individuals reporting rehabilitation through "movement therapy" (i.e., Yoga, Pilates and other groups) were contrasted with individuals who felt they really didn't benefit much at all from these modalities. Three main reasons were found. First, some of the programs did not specifically address all of the main functions of certain core muscles. Secondly, to obtain an advanced proficiency in any of these programs was usually very time consuming and the cost of formal instruction rather expensive. Thirdly, there appeared to be certain genetic factors, which were influential. In themselves, the genetic factors do not appear to cause back pain or strains. However, once a moderate or severe strain has occurred, these genetic factors allow for the "Recurrent Back Strain Syndrome" to both more easily occur and become much more difficult to rehabilitate.

To make a long story short, research theories were formulated. Implementation of these theories rehabilitated my back and stopped the persistent reinjury strains. In 6 months, my back was healthier than I could ever remember it. As stated earlier, from a scientific standpoint, it is very difficult to prove an individual has achieved a healthy back. I felt the best way to prove this to myself would be to work for months in various heavy lifting, blue-collar jobs. This was something I was unable to do on a regular basis after age 22. Mild and moderate strains did occur, but not in the same location that they had for the past 23 years. These mild new location strains proved very useful in being able to more fully evaluate the concepts and theories of Opti-stretch. Also, it demonstrated that my "weak link" had rehabilitated.

The information led to the development of three **<u>screening tests</u>**, which can actually demonstrate that a recognizable problem truly does exist. Any healthy individual can use the Beginning Program screening test. Unfortunately, accurate measurements are more difficult to consistently reproduce. The Intermediate Program screening test allows for very accurate and consistent measurements. However, if you feel any type of stretch while getting into these initial positions in order to start the stretching exercise, this is not acceptable. This was the main reason for developing a Beginning Program. The Advanced Program for Children and Fit Athletes represents stretches, which if they can be comfortably performed, are most consistent with the movements which can be obtained in the "<u>never had back pain</u>" group.

EXPLANATION OF THE SCREENING DIAGNOSTIC TESTS

■ ■ ■

This is the relatively simple part of the book.

One of the most important discoveries of Opti-stretch was the screening tests. In my dealing with recurrent back strain, the problem never made sense from a physiologic standpoint. For the first 10 years the problem was rather straightforward. Sometimes, for 2 to 5 year periods, I could do just about anything most guys my age could do. My back seemed pretty normal until for some reason, it would become reinjured, most commonly by overexertion while lifting.

Various exercise and stretching routines seemed to work quite well and maintained the back in a healthy state for rather long periods of time. However, after age thirty, these same routines became much less effective and the length of time between reinjuries became much shorter. I was always trying new and improved exercise routines in order to rehabilitate my back injuries. They would definitely help heal the acute injury and help me to regain strength, but only to a certain level. Any exertion, beyond that level, would reinjure my back. After my fourth <u>severe</u> strain at age 38, there were seldom 3 months without some type of reinjury. Some of my patients with the diagnosis of "chronic back pain" had better activity levels than I did.

The development of screening exercises, as a result of the Opti-stretch research, was tremendously exciting. For the first time, I could actually see and measure <u>something</u> that was different between myself and those with "never any back pain". Research was then directed at correcting these measurable problems. Once I was able to correct the problem, I was then able to strengthen and condition the muscles to levels consistent with the above average individuals in my age group. There has been only one minor reinjury to that area of the back (which had plagued me for 23 years) during the past six years. Incidentally, the injury occurred not while lifting over 1½ times my body weight but while evaluating a new stretching technique.

Opti-stretch has shown that <u>certain core muscles</u> can clinically exist in a partially healed state for decades. More importantly, even after decades of reinjury, this "weak link" muscle can be nearly 100% or more rehabilitated. In the scientific literature, muscle tissue usually heals in a predictable way. Following injury, most muscles heal in that area of damage to 110%. Severe damage is healed by scar tissue formation. Therefore, this healed area is actually more resistant to strain than other areas of the muscle. A new severe stress delivered to the muscle will cause injury to other areas of the muscle rather than the area that has been healed by scar tissue formation.

Unless specifically tested for, the average individual does not realize that these certain core muscles have not completely healed and exist in this asymptomatic chronically injured muscle state (ACIM). These muscles are essentially asymptomatic and appear to be completely healed but they are not. These asymptomatic chronically injured muscles (ACIMs) possess the following four characteristics (**the 4-T's**): tight, tender, trigger points and a shortened stretch to pain transition. A classic presentation is that an ACIM of the right side of the body will be noticeably tighter than the left side. This asymmetry or unequal movement is easy to detect using the stretching exercises. Over 350 different stretches from multiple sources were carefully reviewed and tested. Only those that were most effective at demonstrating the largest amount of asymmetry for a given specific core muscle (i.e., psoas for the low back and rhomboids for the upper back) were chosen. Several new stretches were designed to accomplish these goals.

These tight muscles (ACIMs) contribute to asymmetry and constitute one of the most striking differences between the recurrent back strain groups and the never had any back pain group. The ACIM muscle is tighter because it is in a mild partially contracted state. This tight muscle will fatigue faster, making it more susceptible to reinjury. The reinjury process then keeps repeating itself given any extremes of activity. The occurrence of this condition represents a major risk factor in the development of the "recurrent back strain syndrome".

Asymmetry of certain core muscles is extremely common in the general population. Many individuals, upon seeing this difference in themselves will say, "everybody is a little different one side compared to the other". This isn't true. Approximately one in every five individuals will have perfect symmetry. However, it is true that the vast majority of over 60 to 80% will have minor differences of less than one inch. Much of this has to do with activities where a dominant arm or leg is consistently utilized. A classic example is a professional baseball pitcher who will have increased range of motion and strength in the pitching arm.

A very important discovery was the demonstration that range of motion asymmetry can exist in the never any back pain group, as long as it is usually less than an inch. Also of note, these individuals were each able to comfortably perform the Standing Squat exercise (exercise #3, Advanced Program for Children and Fit Athletes).

However, in the recurrent back strain group, the difference in stretched range of motion is usually greater than an inch. Sometimes a difference of 6 to 8 inches can be measured. It may sound difficult to believe that a full 2-inch difference in range of motion between the left and right side of the body can go completely unnoticed, let alone an 8-inch difference. However, this degree of range of motion is only used by the body in a limited number of extreme activity levels. When used, it is generally associated with motion of the body. Regarding the core muscles of the body, other joints of the back and extremities can usually be easily recruited to achieve the needed range of motion. Opti-stretch stretching exercises were specifically designed to fix joints in one certain position to prevent this recruitment of other joints. This allows for accurate measurement and assessment of the phenomenon of unequal movement. This is only one of several important reasons why the stretching exercise must be performed as directed.

Like many screening tests in medicine, a positive test suggests there <u>may</u> be a problem, but it doesn't necessarily tell you what is causing the problem. Asymmetry can exist due to extensive use of a dominant limb. While this is usually considered "normal" it can be a factor for injury in the non-dominant limb if certain activities are performed.

There are several **<u>causes of muscle tightening and spasm</u>** on one side. Muscles of the body have 2 completely opposite functions. The first is to contract and move the skeletal structures of the body. The second is to spasm and prevent movement of the musculo-skeletal system in order to allow healing. A partially spasmed muscle ("PSM") or completely spasmed muscle indicates that some type of pathology is causing the muscle to spasm and go into this protective role. It is characterized by an immediate detoning process of the muscle.

The most common cause of a partially spasmed muscle ("PSM") is due to acute injury to the muscle. Another very common cause is due to the formation of an asymptomatic chronically injured muscle (ACIM). The ACIM forms due to a direct strain injury to the muscle tissue itself. However, the healing process has halted for some reason prior to the muscle regaining its optimum health. The second most common problem is tendon shortening of a muscle (i.e., iliopsoas muscle). By optimally toning of the muscle through the Opti-stretch Therapeutic Program or any other program that improves the muscle tone, allows for further strengthening and conditioning of that muscle. When optimum toning, strengthening and conditioning has occurred, even the complex problem of iliopsoas tendon shortening can be over 90% resolved. Unfortunately, there is no known effective way to completely lengthen a tendon, once it has become shortened.

Acute and chronic injuries to joints, ligaments, bone, other tissue, and even an ACIM itself can also cause partial protective spasm of different muscles leading to asymmetry. (This is one reason why other muscles with partial protective spasm must be toned first, before the primary ACIM muscle can be rehabilitated.) These multiple indirect causes lead to the formation of a partially spasmed muscle, which have many of the characteristics of an ACIM muscle. This type of indirect spasm (injury) to muscles falls into the category of **<u>pathologic (malignant) back pain</u>**. There is no way to clinically differentiate between an indirect partial spasm and a direct partial spasm (ACIM). However, with the Opti-stretch therapeutic programs, there is a marked difference in these two types of muscle in how they respond to the program. The indirect partially spasmed muscle usually improves somewhat but often is not totally rehabilitated. In contrast, an ACIM will respond very favorably with a <u>complete healing</u> of the partially spasmed muscle.

Both, an ACIM and other types of partially spasmed muscles ("PSMs") can be present simultaneously in the same muscle. This is the primary reason why rehabilitation of an ACIM, over age 55 to 60, is so difficult. If a common condition such as arthritis of the joint is present, this makes rehabilitation of an ACIM much more difficult and generally less complete. With these types of pathologic problems, sometimes only a 10 to 20% improvement can be realistically expected. The good news is that even the small amount of improvement can markedly improve an individuals' activity level and quality of life. In working with many individuals over the age of 55, complete toning of the muscles has been extremely difficult due to joint arthritis, normal aging processes of the muscle and other chronic conditions. This is a good reason for individuals to learn Opti-stretch before the age of 35 and definitely before age 50, if at all possible.

The Opti-stretch therapeutic program was specifically designed for ACIMs. If this very specific condition exists, quite spectacular results can occur. However, many are finding noticeable benefit depending on the pathological cause of the "PSMs" such as certain types of herniated discs. The goal of Opti-stretch is to return muscle tone and help correct asymmetry. Even small improvements in muscle tone can decrease this imbalance and improve the health of various core muscle groups.

In addition to the importance of demonstrating unequal or asymmetric movement between the left and the right side of the body, there is a certain minimum range of motion needed by the core muscles in order to safely lift heavy objects. By being able to distribute the lifting force equally throughout the legs and back, helps protect the commonly injured area of the psoas muscle. This concept is much more complex and needs to be tailored to the individual body type. These genetically-controlled, body type factors ("BTFs") such as height, gender, frame size, muscle mass, and morphism have to be taken into consideration. It requires a good working knowledge of anatomy and physiology. Again, the "Standing Squat" exercise was extremely helpful in determining minimal range of motion for certain core muscles of the back and helping to differentiate asymmetry which can be due to excess use of a dominant limb. If you have to grab the object to bring yourself down to the proper straight-back lifting position, an additional 20 to 30 pounds of force are placed on the psoas complex.

Asymmetry of range of motion can easily be determined by the average individual by simply performing the screening tests and measuring the results. For a more complete evaluation, an instructor in Opti-stretch with more extensive anatomy and physiology knowledge is necessary. The screening diagnostic tests are designed for anyone who is healthy. Those who are over age 40 should have permission from their doctor, before even starting the screening tests. This helps to insure adequate health, so that no untoward event will occur.

THOSE THAT ALREADY HAVE A HEALTHY BACK.

The screening diagnostic tests document not only if the body moves symmetrically, but also gives an accurate and reproducible measurement of the stretched range of motion of the joints and muscles. Should an accident occur such as a car wreck or bad fall, recovery of this stretched range of motion is extremely important for <u>complete recovery</u> or maximum expected recovery. This knowledge can be invaluable in knowing when the individual has completely recovered the preexisting muscle tone and can safely go on to full strengthening and conditioning of the muscles. Also, loss of this stretched range of motion is a major factor in the aging process. There are multiple reasons for this process. However, the longer an individual can maintain this optimum range of motion, generally the more activities they can participate in, and the younger they will feel.

CHILDREN.

This is for the Dr. Mom's. Opti-stretch research shows over 95% of all healthy 3 to 5 year olds who are close to ideal body weight can perform the Advanced Program for Children and Fit Athletes. Moreover, this absolute stretched range of motion is extremely uniform for all individuals in this age group regardless of the body type factors ("BTFs"). Opti-stretch has determined this range of motion to be a "gold standard". Range of motion beyond this level can be helpful for special activities (i.e., gymnastics and martial arts). However, excess range of motion beyond the "gold standard" does not appear to significantly help in rehabilitating a "bad back" or in preserving a healthy back throughout life.

Once documented at this age, every 6 months or yearly the screening test should be repeated to assure there is no change. If there is a change due to a developing specific body type, the decrease in range of motion should be completely symmetrical. Opti-stretch research suggests that many of the initial injuries actually occur in childhood, which then later predispose the individual to recurrent back strain in puberty and early adulthood.

By age 6, gender difference and the 12 to 20% of the population with hyperflexibility start to be clinically manifested. It has been known for hundreds of years that individuals with hyperflexibility have at least the same or even a higher incidence of back pain. That is the reason why certain levels of flexibility have never been promoted in modern medicine beyond what is concluded to be the " normal voluntary range of motion" as measured by most physicians. "Stretched range of motion", in the past, has been far too variable, problematic, and time consuming to be clinically useful except in certain limb and shoulder injuries. Remember, absolute range of motion is not the key.

Asymmetry is the key to look for. Even then, certain small amounts of asymmetry are considered to be normal in certain individuals. The Intermediate Screening Tests will accurately detect the majority of important core-muscle asymmetry problems, even in the hyperflexible or double-jointed individuals.

Another valuable use of this knowledge is determining when an adolescent can return to full activity. Almost every kid crashes a bicycle or gets banged up. Frequently, some kids will reinjure themselves if allowed to return to full activity too soon. If they are comfortably able to perform the Advanced Program, there is less chance of reinjury when returning to full activity. By comparing to previous test measurement, this will help Dr. Mom to evaluate whether any residual muscular injury of a core muscle has occurred.

MEASURING AND DETECTING ACIMs. (NOW IT'S TIME TO GET STARTED)

Little is needed to get started. You'll need this book and a ruler or tape measure. Then, find a comfortable carpet or exercise mat. Consider this book as a workbook that should be written in. If you are one of the many that just can't bring themselves to write in books, you will need some paper and a pencil.

Certain very important concepts are necessary to understand in order to prevent injury. Most important is that you **must not over-stretch**! Stretched range of motion is nothing more than applying a certain force to the muscles which possess visco-elastic properties. The amount of force is referred to as the intensity of stretch. However, if the force is applied too rapidly, in a jerking fashion or with too much intensity, stretch receptors within muscles, joints and tendons will detect this as a noxious (injurious) stimulus. Muscles then reflexively contract to protect the body from injury. When this happens, even more stress is placed on certain muscle tissues, which can increase the chance of injury.

Opti-stretch research has demonstrated that the majority of individuals over-stretch. This is especially common in children and adolescents. Most adults have not tried to stretch their muscles since they were an adolescent and participating in sports. The above mentioned groups will just force the muscle until it hurts. Past the age of 35 and if asymptomatic chronically injured muscles (ACIMs) are present, this over-stretching significantly increases the chance of injury. Even micro-injury can predispose a young athlete to a more serious strain during a game. Incidentally, individuals that overstretch do not like to perform stretching exercises and are less likely to do so when older.

Most books dealing with stretching recommend gently increasing the stretch until the individual feels moderate discomfort. With the screening test, an individual can choose either a mild or moderate intensity of stretch. The specific point between mild and moderate is usually the safest. (Note that it is extremely important not to bounce). It is also very important that the same intensity of stretch is used for both sides of the body. This is especially true if a mild intensity of stretch is performed. A mild intensity of stretch on one side and a moderate intensity of stretch on the other side will narrow the differences and decrease the accuracy while measuring stretched range of motion. The stretch must be held comfortably for at least 5 to 10 seconds and then measured.

Stretched range of motion involves determining how far the relaxed muscle will allow a joint to move in a given plane of motion. Normal, non-stretched range of motion is determined by how far an individual can move a joint by either voluntarily contracting or relaxing certain muscles. In clinical medicine, this is measured with a goniometer in degrees of joint movement. An indirect way to measure stretched range of motion is both easier and more accurate for most individuals. Opti-stretch screening tests use the distance between 2 determined anatomical points to measure range of motion (say touching the nose to the knee). It is very easy to determine and remember when your nose was 3 inches away from your knee, compared to now being only 1 inch away. Likewise, it is easy to determine even small amounts of progress. Measurement with a goniometer is complex and time consuming. A great deal of normal anatomy has to be understood before the results are both accurate and reproducible. (Unfortunately, this type of 2-point measurement of Opti-stretch does lead to problems both in comparing different individuals and to be able to scientifically publish data. In my opinion, the simplicity and value to the individual who wants to accomplish certain Opti-stretch goals is well worth it.)

The next most common cause of injury is that our minds are goal oriented. A very common problem is to say "I can put my nose on my knee" or "with a little effort, I can do that". Through a number of complex mechanisms, the brain will attempt to help you achieve this goal. Unfortunately, this can often lead to muscle strain (especially in a poorly toned muscle). To avoid injury due to focusing on a distance, shut your eyes after detecting the "first sensation of stretch" (see below) and focus entirely on what sensations the stretch receptors are telling you. Many prefer just partially closing the eyes so that the distant point is somewhat obscured. **Never decide in advance or actively focus on what point you want to achieve!** Focus only on the information that the stretch receptors of your body are indicating as to the intensity of the stretch.

Everyone is different in their own opinion of what is mild discomfort and when it becomes moderate discomfort. For example, the sensation of moderate discomfort for an 8-year-old boy and a 28-year-old NFL football player are not even remotely the same. In future chapters, you will learn how to determine accurately these levels for yourself.

Also, there are "extreme individuals" who push any activity to its most extreme level. Therefore, a maximum intensity of force that one can deliver to a muscle and still avoid injury is discussed later. Once you can learn and interpret the different sensations produced by your various stretch receptors (i.e., muscle, tendon and ligament), you will learn first hand how complex the muscular organ system of the body really is. You can then appreciate the impact fatigue, anxiety, stress, illness and various cyclical changes can have on the muscles in the body. This knowledge is referred to as the first aid part of the Opti-stretch program.

Most of the stretching exercises in this book show two positions, the "start of the stretch" and the "gold standard" level of stretch. The start of the stretch demonstrates where most average individuals will feel the "first sensation of stretch". The "first sensation of stretch" is a very important concept in Opti-stretch research. Any movement, prior to this position should produce no sensation of stretching in any muscle group. Also, a trained professional can objectively detect this precise point in an individual, by feeling the change in resistance of muscles as the individual approaches this point. This is very exciting for several reasons. First, many large groups of individuals will have nearly the identical point as their "first sensation of stretch". From a scientific standpoint, it is important to know that a professional can detect very precisely this point for research purposes. In the past, electronic sensors were placed on the muscle. Unfortunately for several muscles, like the psoas muscle, the location of these deep core muscles in the body does not allow for placement of electronic sensors and other experimental probes.

Next, in normal and healthy individuals without any acute injuries, this point is very symmetrical when comparing the left and right sides of the body. Even individuals who have tight ACIMs up to 8 inches will still have normal symmetry for their "first sensation of stretch" on both the left and right sides. However, with acute injury to the muscle, this point will be altered and occur sooner helping to differentiate chronic and acute injuries. Scientifically, this is very valuable information. Also, it is important knowledge for everyone. This knowledge can serve as important first aid information. Awareness of even mild acute injuries can allow individuals to adequately protect the muscle. Frequently, these mild injuries are reinjured and converted to a much more serious strain injury.

Unfortunately due to space in the book, the second photo is usually the "gold standard". This stretched range of motion, for the majority of people, appears quite extreme. It is very important to realize two things. Most adults with documented very healthy backs **cannot** achieve this "gold standard" range of motion. Also, individuals with very bad backs can easily achieve this level (if they are genetically hyperflexible). Unfortunately, for some individuals with a long history of ACIMs, they must achieve this level before the chronically injured muscle can become completely toned. The "gold standard" can then be considered a stopping point or accomplished goal. Achieving range of motion beyond this level does not appear to significantly help in the rehabilitation process of ACIMs.

When measuring on the screening diagnostic tests, you can detect ACIMs even in the mild discomfort intensity level if you pay attention to only the stretch receptors. The screening tests should be performed at this level in older individuals and those with severe ACIMs to avoid strain injuries to these sensitive muscles. This program focuses on important core muscles that are seldom used daily and are the most easily injured with excessive activities. Because you are using highly leveraged stretches specifically on the core muscles that have chronic injuries, an acute injury can easily occur if you are not careful. In the Opti-stretch Therapeutic Programs, you will stay at the mild intensity of stretch for the first two months or until the muscles are toned to a level where they can tolerate, without injury, a higher intensity of stretch.

After detecting the "first sensation of stretch", which is the start of a mild discomfort sensation, slowly continue the stretch until a different sensation occurs. Stop, open your eyes and measure the distance between the two reference points. Most stretches are named according to these reference points making these points easy to remember (i.e., Sitting Nose to Knee). Next, record the distance (the easiest is in inches). A very common error is not to write this information down. Most people don't want to record this level because they think their own level is just too bad to record. Others think, "I'll just remember it". (This is extremely difficult when the point has been gradually changing over 6 months.) This recorded information is extremely valuable, as previously mentioned, for the purpose of rehabilitation should a severe accident occur. Having worked in the field of Physical Therapy, many individuals are determined as being back to "average normal" range of motion when their own previous level of normal has not yet been obtained. This can lead to problems in the future.

Recording the results can serve as an important reference point in your life and can be followed to see how you are progressing or at least staying the same. Each program should be measured 3 times so you can pick which set of numbers best represent your starting point. Remember, the normal adult aging process will continue to decrease the stretched range of motion. The longer you maintain this level (even if it is somewhat limited), the more activities you can participate in as you age. Your doctor may even consider you as "younger than stated age".

Everyone except children should start with the Beginning Program screening stretches. A good idea is to do this beginning screening test on different days for 3 days. Record your best results. Next proceed to the Intermediate Program. These are more complex stretches. (Many will feel they are past the "first sensation of stretch" just getting into the starting position of a particular stretching exercise. If you happen to be one of these individuals, stop and proceed to the upper back and neck screening exercises. Chances are high that you will benefit from the Opti-stretch Therapeutic Program which is presented later in this book.)

Next, attempt the upper back and neck screening diagnostic stretches from the Intermediate Program and record your results. Remember that neck muscles are extremely fragile compared with the lower back muscles. Extra caution in attempting these screening diagnostic stretches is very important in order to avoid a strain.

If able to successfully pass the Intermediate test to the "gold standard", "children and fit athletes" can then proceed to the Advanced Program. An extra word of caution is necessary for the exercise called the "Standing Squat". This stretch is comfortably and routinely performed by individuals in their 60's and 70's in many 3rd world nations. Prior to the 1980's this stretch was routinely used in the medical profession to demonstrate subtle alterations in blood flow, which were useful in detecting certain right heart murmurs. If you cannot comfortably perform this stretch and then try to force yourself into this position, very significant alterations in blood flow can occur. Even a healthy individual can feel dizzy and even pass out. If you have certain abnormalities or disease processes, this can be extremely dangerous.

Anyone over the age of 40 not only should have a physical exam by their physician. They should also have a qualified spotter (assistant) for the first couple of times. Remember that serious consequences can occur with any medical problems and especially those with cerebral aneurysm, high blood pressure, heart disease and deep vein thrombosis.

The above guidelines are identical for the "Bridge" stretching exercise. They are designed for children ages 3 to 5 because they can be fun for the children, while at the same time evaluating multiple joints and muscles which are important in lifting heavy objects and maintaining a healthy back. Because over 95% of children ages 3 to 5 can comfortably perform these advanced exercises, this serves as an excellent guideline of normalcy. In first world nations, the percentage of individuals who can comfortably perform these stretching exercises falls by 10-20% each decade. By age 50, this rate has fallen to a low percentage of the population. However, there are individuals over age 50 that can perform these advanced stretches to the level of the "gold standard". All these individuals considered themselves to have very healthy backs. If these stretches can be comfortably performed throughout adolescence and adulthood, Opti-stretch research suggests this may be a good way to preserve the optimum function of the spine. The one possible exception is in the hyperflexible group of individuals. A chapter is dedicated to this group who are experiencing recurrent back pain.

Asymmetry of more than 2 inches is frequently found in individuals with "recurrent back strain syndrome". When the asymmetry is an inch or less, the chance of "recurrent strains" in a single location are diminished unless underlying pathology is present. Having had the opportunity to evaluate even world class athletes, few can perform all the stretches to the level of the "gold standard". However, the majority can usually come within 3 to 5 inches of this level very comfortably.

If you can comfortably pass all of the screening tests (Beginning, Intermediate and Advanced), you have successfully completed the major goals of the Opti-stretch Program. Thank Mother Nature, record your results and consider completing the Opti-stretch Therapeutic Program prior to age 30. It is helpful in understanding the optimum function of the muscles and serves as great first aid knowledge should an injury occur. After age 35, when muscles start changing due to the normal aging process, this knowledge will be extremely valuable. The only other recommendation is to find an enjoyable sport or activity to preserve this stretched range of motion for life.

For those who have the symptoms of "recurrent back strains" or have asymmetry of the body of over an inch, this book is dedicated to you. My sincere wishes are that you may find this knowledge as beneficial as I did in helping me to stop the process of recurrent strains (a major problem in my low back and a less severe area in my upper back).

QUESTIONS AND ANSWERS

SHOULD EVERYONE TRY OPTI-STRETCH?

Everyone who is healthy enough to try the stretching exercises should take advantage of this knowledge. First, if there is no problem, the information serves as an excellent reference as to what your normal range of motion is, should a significant injury occur. Second, by completing the program a great deal of knowledge is gained about the musculo-skeletal system of your body. Especially in later life, this knowledge provides first aid information for avoiding muscular injury and detecting even minimal and mild strain injuries. Once a strain appears to have healed, Opti-stretch can detect whether a partially injured muscular problem remains. Third, if due to illness or other conditions a problem with risk factors does occur, improved toning of the muscles can help an individual to avoid significant strains to those muscles.

WHAT IS THE DEFINITION OF ACTIVITY LEVEL?

Activity level is an important concept in assessing back health but is very difficult to quantify scientifically. The minimum independent functioning of an individual are defined as the Activities of Daily Living (<u>ADL</u>). Individuals with "bad backs" due to "recurrent back strain syndromes" will experience very few back strains if this activity level is <u>strictly</u> maintained. However, if their situation in life changes to where they are required to maintain a higher activity level, the ACIMs will frequently become reinjured.

Even blue-collar workers who can lift significant amounts of weight all day without difficulty can still have ACIMs and serious risk factors for back strain. If they change jobs to where lifting from uneven surfaces and twisting while lifting is required, they often find their "recurrent back strain" will flair up.

Testing of the back for strength and conditioning can be done but is very problematic and potentially dangerous for certain age groups. Currently, there is no excellent scientific gold standard of activity level measurement. The general concept of "run, jump, climb, work, play and keep up with the other kids your age", is a valuable concept. Opti-stretch stretching exercises appear to be an excellent way of predicting a healthy back.

Should everyone achieve the Opti-stretch "gold standard" level of range-of-motion?

The "gold standard" level of tone allows excellent general function of the core muscles. Toning beyond that level does not appear to significantly improve back health. If you were a healthy 3 to 5 year old, you once possessed this range of motion. (That is why the majority of individuals can obtain this level with a sufficient amount of effort over a 6-month period of time.)

Remember, many world class athletes with very healthy backs have range of motion somewhat less than the "gold standard". However, they are usually very symmetrical. Also, they are usually very close to the "gold standard". There are certain body types that can have a fairly limited range of motion, yet have very healthy backs. The concept is valuable for those with severe recurrent back problems to set realistic goals and be able to recognize when the back pain is due to a cause other than muscle strain.

Remember these are basic guidelines. The optimum range of motion is partially genetically determined and is dependent on multiple factors. Optimum tone of your own muscles is the most important goal no matter what your range of motion. Tone is defined as a measured amount of range of motion beginning from the "first sensation of stretch" given a certain quantity of force and not exceeding a certain level of discomfort. Optimum is somewhere between too little and too much. Without scientific measuring devices, stretched range of motion is currently one of the better indicators of tone. Hopefully, in the near future, we will be able to more accurately determine what is the "normal" range of motion for a specific body type. Opti-stretch has contributed to this goal in being able to easily screen for double-jointed individuals and genetic hyperflexibility.

Notes

_____

_____

_____

_____

_____

_____

STEP #1 OF THE OPTI-STRETCH CHALLENGE (SCREENING TESTS)

■ ■ ■

You are now ready to take the Opti-stretch screening tests (which are the exercises in each program). If you are medically qualified, have no current injury or pain and in the "recurrent back strain" group or the "never any back pain" group, you are set. One other group may be considered. Previous herniated disc patients with recurrent back pain may consider the screening test if cleared for regular activity and at least six months out from a disc injury.

For safety and efficiency, the majority of stretches are performed in the sitting position. All Opti-stretch Beginning and Intermediate stretching exercises are specifically designed so the stretching force can immediately be released. (This is why the Opti-stretch therapeutic stretch-receptor-lengthening technique must not be used on any other stretching exercises.)

Find a comfortable carpet or an exercise mat. The Beginning Stretching Exercises were designed for even advanced age groups. You can find the Beginning Screening Test in the next chapter and the corresponding worksheets in the Appendix. Any difference of more than one to two inches on the left side versus the right side is considered to be a major risk factor.

If you can comfortably get into the desired stretching exercise position, slowly and gently proceed to where you first feel a stretch of any kind. This "first sensation of stretch" will normally persist for at least 2 more inches of stretch and by definition is the range of <u>mild</u> stretch. At this point, another level of discomfort will appear (defined as <u>moderate</u>). Normally, this level of discomfort will persist identically until another <u>moderately-severe</u> level of discomfort will be felt (which is normally at least another couple of inches). The transition from mild to moderate is the best stopping point (especially if you are over age 45). Only if you have extensive experience with stretching, should the moderate discomfort limit be explored. Record your results.

Upon recording the results of the Beginning Program screening tests, most can proceed to the Intermediate Program. If there is any sensation of stretch while carefully getting into the starting position, immediately stop. Most can safely proceed to the upper back and neck screening exercises. Record your results for these exercises in the Appendix.

If any risk factors are detected, you may be in a high-risk category for "recurrent back strain" to reoccur. A common scenario is that if the muscles of the right side of the low back are tight, the right side of the upper back will be tight and the left side of the neck will be tight. You can easily confirm that the muscles are tender by simply massaging the muscles on each side. A great way to convince yourself is to get a deep muscle massage of the back and neck by a licensed massage therapist or someone knowledgeable about massage. Chances are high that they will confirm that you have tender and tight muscles with knots (trigger points) <u>on the same side</u> of the body that you found the tight muscles using the Opti-stretch screening test.

A common misconception at this point is that "everyone has a left or right side of the body that is a little different". This statement is partially accurate. In fact, the overwhelming majority (approximately 80%) of the population has this problem to one degree or another. However, 20% of the population does not. The majority of these individuals are also in the "never had any back pain" group. In fact, there is a high probability that you don't even know someone in the "never had any back pain" group who enjoys a high to extremely high activity level.

<u>Remember</u> that the Opti-stretch therapeutic programs were specifically designed for individuals with "recurrent back strain" and demonstrable risk factors, in order to correct these risk factors. The closer that you can get the left side of the body functioning like the right side of the body, the less difficulty you will have with "recurrent back strain".

If the Beginning and Intermediate screening stretches seem easy and no risk factors can be detected, go to the Opti-stretch Advanced Program. Easy completion of the Advanced Program screening test with no indication that one side of the body moves different than the other, means that you have passed Step 3 of the Opti-stretch Challenge. Chances are very high that you possess a healthy back. The goal for most at this level is a Maintenance Program. A yearly check is one option to make sure no risk factors have developed. Some individuals in their 50's and 70's can easily perform most of these stretching exercises. If you happen to be age 75 or older, and can still comfortably perform the Advanced Program screening test, I would enjoy hearing from you. There are many individuals who are extremely active at age 85 (i.e., still continue to snow ski). For the baby-boomer generation, this is both a realistic and desirable goal. Opti-stretch can be a helpful tool in attaining this goal.

Make certain to record your results. While 20% of the population appears almost immune from common back strain, serious accidents or injuries can happen. Data generated from Opti-stretch can be extremely valuable in knowing when you are back to 100% following something similar to a car accident or a broken bone.

Record results on the various worksheets located in the Appendix!

OPTI-STRETCH
BEGINNING PROGRAM

■ ■ ■

If you had any significant tightness or problems with the Screening Test Stretches, or if you are over age 45, you should consider starting at the beginning level. This is both an easier and safer level to start out at. Upon completion of the Beginning Program, you should be able to comfortably get into the starting position of each of the exercises in the Intermediate Therapeutic Program.

1. **Kneeling Chest to Knee**
2. **Supine Knee to Chest**
3. **Supine Knee to Chest with Nose to Knee**
4. **Supine Hip Hike**
5. **Supine Knee to Cross Chest**
6. **Supine Straight Knee to Nose**
7. **Sitting Knees to Floor – (Butterfly)**
8. **Supine Both Knees to Chest**

NOTE:
The Beginning Program will be used both as a
screening test and with the Therapeutic Technique.

---

1. Kneeling Chest to Knee – Erector Spinae Stretch

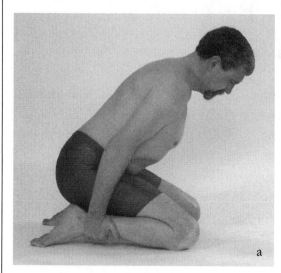 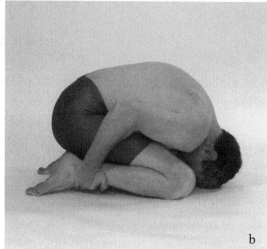

a.   b

a. Wide stance kneeling starting position. Toes should be pointing straight back. Buttocks should be resting on the heels.
b. Fetal position curl. Attempt to place the chest gently to the thighs and forehead between the knees.

Notes:
1. This is a relaxing position to begin warming-up the low back. It can be eliminated if time is short.
2. This is the same as the "Kneeling Nose to Floor". The major difference is that you should not try to flex the neck to the floor. This can be too strenuous for certain individuals.
3. This again should be a comfortable warm-up stretch. If you find it uncomfortable do not perform this stretch.

Risk factors:
1. If unable to get the nose 4 inches above the knees, this suggests a possible limitation in normal range of motion for flexion of the spine.
2. If unable to comfortably place the chest onto the knees suggests there may be some difficulty in performing the stretching exercise of "Sitting Nose to Knee" (Figure Four).

2. SUPINE KNEE TO CHEST – HAMSTRING STRETCH

3. SUPINE KNEE TO CHEST WITH NOSE TO KNEE – HAMSTRING AND NECK STRETCH

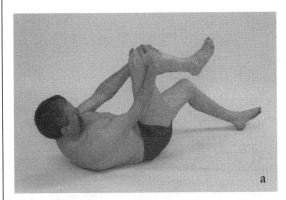

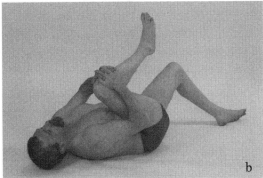

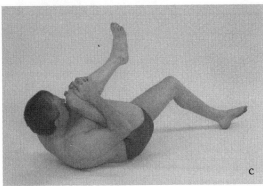

a. Start in the supine position (lying on back). Grab the right knee and start to bring it toward the chest.
b. Using the strength of the arms, bring the knee as close to the chest as possible. Do not attempt to touch the nose to the knee.
c. This is a separate exercise of slowly touching the nose to knee. It is used for measurement. Avoid, if you have any neck problems.

Notes
1. Repeat the same process for the left leg.
2. When comfortable with the "Knee to Chest", measure with the "Nose to Knee" stretch. Upon being able to touch the "Nose to Knee" you are ready for some of the Intermediate Therapeutic Program.

4. SUPINE HIP HIKE – QUADRATUS LUMBORUM STRETCH EXERCISE

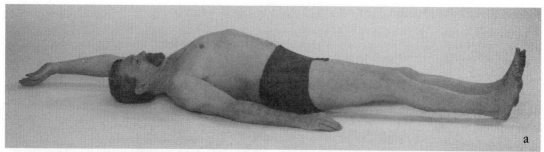

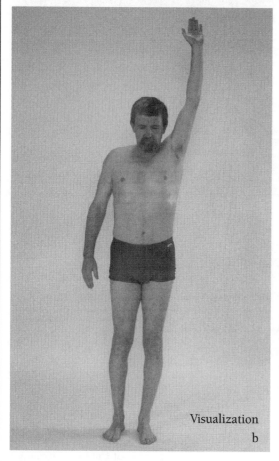

Visualization
b

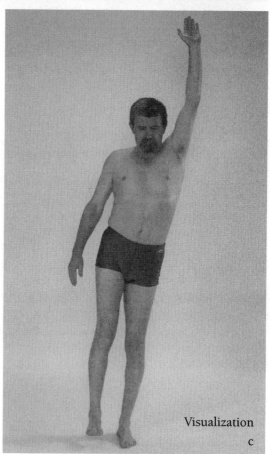

Visualization
c

a. In the supine position, extend the left arm overhead. Then hike the right hip up toward the right shoulder.
b. More easily visualized in the standing position.
c. With the left arm extended hike the right hip.

Notes:
1. Repeat the process for the right arm and left hip.
2. The major stretch is in the low back (a muscle known as the quadratus lumborum). A fair amount of slow gradual hike of the hip is necessary to feel the optimum stretch and contraction of the quadratus lumborum muscle. Remember to bring the hip up slowly and evenly.
3. The stretch should feel slightly different depending which arm is placed overhead. Example: right arm – right hip or left arm – left hip.

5. Supine Knee to Cross Chest – Pyriformis Stretch

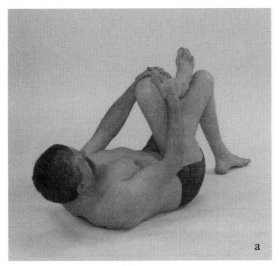 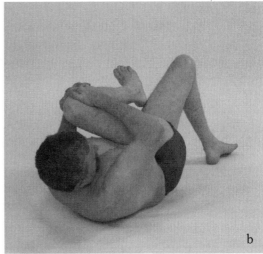

a.   In the supine position, grab the right knee. The right heel should be placed on the outside edge of the left thigh.

b.   Bring the right knee toward the cross chest or the left axilla.

Notes:

1.   Repeat the process for the left knee.

2.   This puts a stretch on the right buttocks muscles called the major hip flexors. The pyriformis muscle is part of this group.

3.   Initially, be very slow and careful with this group of muscles, as these major hip flexors can be very tender and sensitive to this stretch.

4.   The head does not need to be raised, if there are any neck problems.

6. SUPINE STRAIGHT KNEE TO NOSE

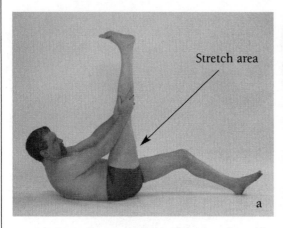

Stretch area

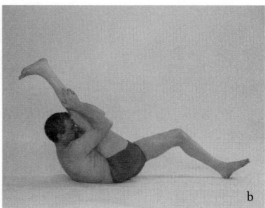

a. In the supine position, grab either the calf or the thigh (preferably the calf) of the right leg. Keep the knee straight.
b. Attempt to bring the knee to the nose.

Notes:
1. Repeat for the left leg.
2. This is the stretch that will allow you to start into the Intermediate Therapeutic Exercises with "Sitting Nose to Knee" (Figure Four).
3. This is a very good exercise to use to help determine the force intensity, which will cause a moderate-discomfort level of stretch.
4. The nose to knee should be within about a foot before progressing to the "Sitting Nose to Knee" position.
5. Remember, it is important to keep the knee fully extended.
6. Another way to do the exercise is to leave the knee partially bent. Then slowly straighten the knee to perform the stretch. This is an excellent exercise for quadriceps strengthening.

7. SITTING KNEES TO FLOOR – (BUTTERFLY)

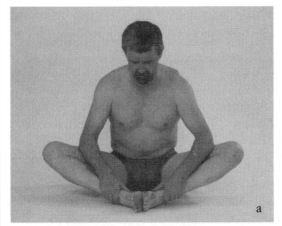

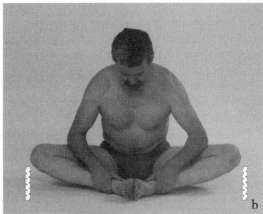

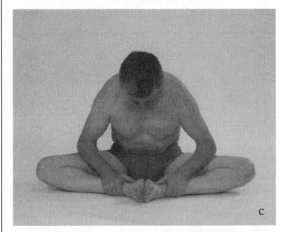

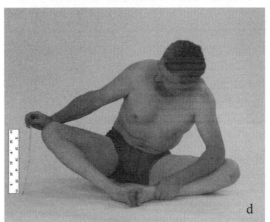

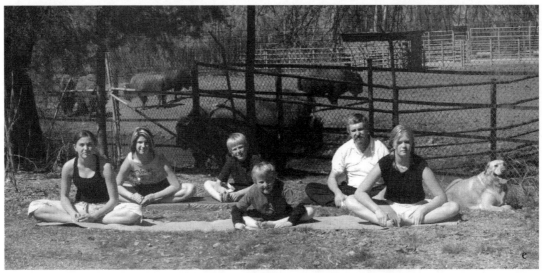

7. SITTING KNEES TO FLOOR (CONTINUED)

a. In the sitting position bring the soles of the feet together. Grasp the ankles and rest the elbows on the thighs close to the knees.

b. Another useful measurement is to measure the height of the knees off the floor using only the strength of the arms to bring both knees close to the floor. Relax and measure the height off the floor for the knees.

c. Exert pressure on the thighs by using the elbows. Slowly push the legs flat on the floor if possible. For this position, this is an anatomically delineated stretch (you can only go so far before the floor stops you).

d. Next, exert pressure on the left thigh with the left elbow until the leg is flat on the floor. With the right hand on the right knee gently stretch the groin area. In some individuals, a definite difference in the sensation of the stretch is felt for different legs. While in this position, measure the height of the knee off the floor for each leg.

e. In most children this is a very comfortable stretch. In many athletic adult males while even using the force of the elbows, the knees are usually 2 1/2 inches off the floor.

Notes:
1. This is an important stretch for several reasons. First, it can be accurately measured. Second, the groin muscles are very sensitive to being overstretched. Comparison with the force used for stretching the hamstring muscles will allow the individual to learn how various muscles groups respond differently to various amounts of force that are placed on them.
2. Knees should be at least 4 inches from the floor before proceeding on to the other Intermediate stretches.

8. Supine Both Knees to Chest

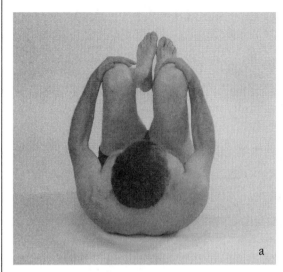
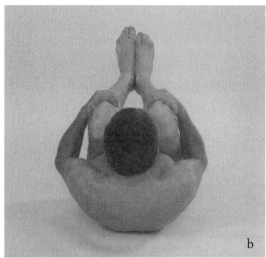

a.   Grab both knees at the same time.

b.   Attempt to bring the knees to the chest.

Notes:

1. This is a slightly advanced exercise and should be practiced only after becoming comfortable with the "Supine Knee to Chest".
2. This stretching exercise can put a great deal of stress on the low back so be very cautious to perform the exercise carefully and slowly.
3. The head can rest comfortably on the floor or a pillow if the stretch bothers the shoulders or neck.

OPTI-STRETCH
INTERMEDIATE PROGRAM

■ ■ ■

1. Kneeling Nose to Floor
2. Sitting Nose to Knee – (Figure Four)
3. Supine Straight Knee to Nose
4. Sitting Knees to Floor – (Butterfly)
5. Sitting Knee to Cross Chest
6. Kneeling wide Stance Pelvis to Floor
7. Kneeling Elbows Back to Floor
8. Prone Twisting Crawl
9. Sitting cheerleader – Nose to Knee
10. Sitting cheerleader – Elbow to Ankle
11. Sitting cheerleader – Hip to Cross Knee
12. Kneeling Narrow Stance Pelvis to Floor – (Cobra)
13. Rhomboid pull
14. Finger Touch
15. Chin to Shoulder
16. Chin Backwards
17. Ear to Shoulder
18. Straight Arm Ear to Shoulder
19. Chin to Chest
20. Ear to Axilla (Armpit)

NOTE:
Intermediate Program to be used both as screening
tests and with The Therapeutic Technique.

---

1. KNEELING NOSE TO FLOOR – ERECTOR SPINAE STRETCH

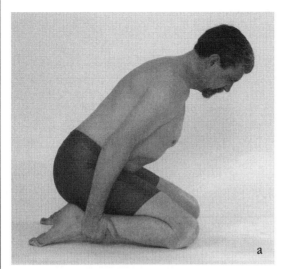
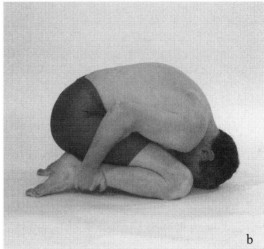

a.   Wide stance kneeling position to start. Toes should be pointing straight back. Buttocks should be resting on the heels.

b.   Fetal position curl. Attempt to place the chest gently to the knees. Attempt to place the forehead between the knees.

Notes:

1.   This is a relaxing position to begin warming-up the low back. It can be eliminated if time is short. It allows detection of any injury to the erector spinae muscles.
2.   Those with neck problems should be extremely careful not to overflex the neck.
3.   This again should be a comfortable warm-up stretch. If you find it uncomfortable do not perform this stretch.

Risk factors:

1.   If unable to get the nose 4 inches above the knees, this suggests a possible limitation in normal range of motion for flexion of the spine.
2.   If unable to comfortably place the chest onto the knees suggests there may be some difficulty in performing the stretching exercise of "Sitting Nose to Knee" (Figure Four).

2. SITTING NOSE TO KNEE – (FIGURE FOUR) – HAMSTRING STRETCH

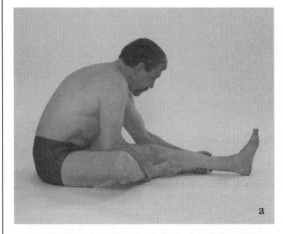

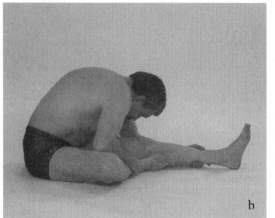

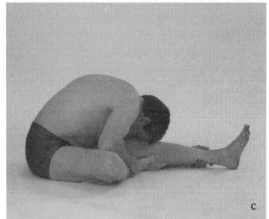

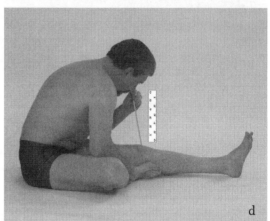

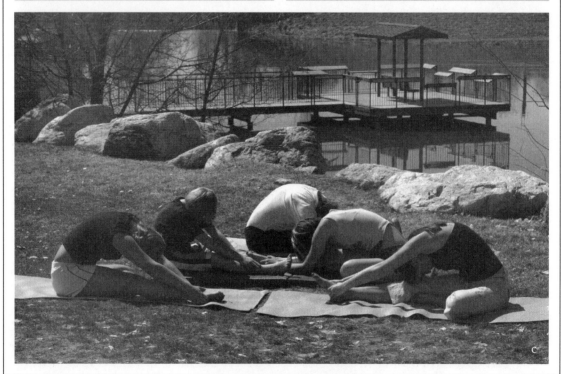

2. SITTING NOSE TO KNEE – (FIGURE FOUR) (CONTINUED)

a. Sit with the left knee extended. The right knee is bent with the arch of the foot touching the inside of the knee. Note the position so it can be duplicated on the right side.

b. Slowly attempt to touch the nose to the knee. When the nose is two inches above the knee, this is the start of the excellent position. The majority of 6-year-olds can obtain this position.

c. Maximum stretch is the chin to the knee and holding the left foot. This is an example of an anatomically delimited stretch for a given stretch or position. If the stretch is performed in the standing position even greater stretch could be delivered to the hamstring muscles by extending the head past the knee. This is also much more dangerous of a stretch.

d. Measure the precise distance with a flexible tape measure or piece of string on each side.

Note: If unable to even sit comfortably in the (a) position, then it is important to start with the "Supine Straight Knee to Nose" stretching exercise [Exercise: 3(a) and 3(b)] until the sitting position becomes comfortable.

Risk factors for Back Pain
1. More than one inch in measured difference between the left and right side.
2. Inability to get into the "Sitting Nose to Knee" position comfortably.

3. SUPINE STRAIGHT KNEE TO NOSE

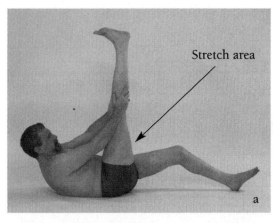
Stretch area
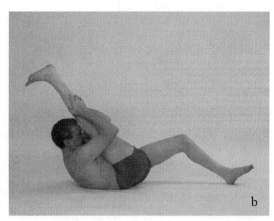

a

b

a. In the supine position, grab either the calf or the thigh (preferably the calf) of the right leg. Keep the knee straight.

b. Attempt to bring the knee to the nose.

Notes:
1. Repeat for the left leg.
2. This is the stretch that will allow you to start into the Intermediate Therapeutic Exercises with "Sitting Nose to Knee" (Figure Four).
3. This is a very good exercise to use for helping to determine the force intensity, which will cause a moderate discomfort level of stretch.
4. The nose to knee should be within about a foot before progressing to the "Sitting Nose to Knee" position.
5. Remember, it is important to keep the knee fully extended.
6. Another way to do the exercise is to leave the knee partially bent. Then slowly straighten the knee to perform the stretch. This is an excellent exercise for quadriceps strengthening.

4. Sitting knee to floor – (Butterfly)

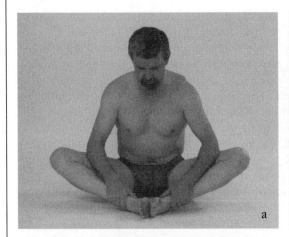
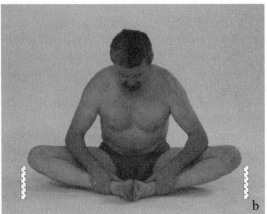

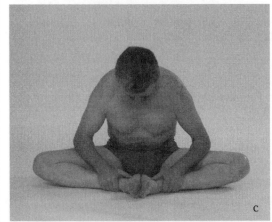
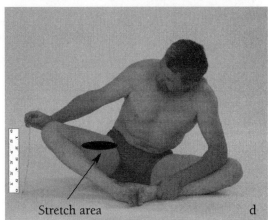

Stretch area

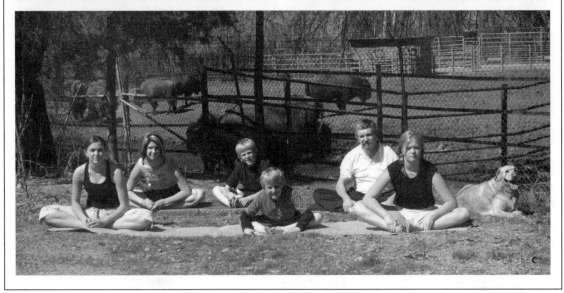

4. SITTING KNEE TO FLOOR – (BUTTERFLY) (CONTINUED)

a. In the sitting position bring the soles of the feet together. Grasp the ankles and rest the elbows on the thighs close to the knees.

b. This is the level which many excellent male athletes can obtain.

c. Exert pressure on the thighs by using the elbows. Slowly push the legs flat on the floor if possible. For this position, this is an anatomically delineated stretch (you can only go so far before the floor stops you). If unable to obtain this position measure as in figure (b).

d. Next, exert pressure on the left thigh with the left elbow until the leg is flat on the floor. With the right hand on the right knee gently stretch the groin area. In some individuals, a definite difference in the sensation of the stretch is felt for different legs. While in this position, measure the height of the knee off the floor for each leg.

e. In most children this is a very comfortable stretch. In many athletic adult males while even using the force of the elbows, the knees are usually $2^1/2$ inches off the floor.

Notes: This is an important stretch for several reasons. First, it can be accurately measured. Second, these groin muscles are very sensitive to being overstretched. Comparison with the (Figure Four) stretch for stretching the hamstring muscles will allow the individual to learn how various muscles groups respond differently to various amounts of force that are placed on them.

Risk factors:

1. As seen in figure (4-b), if the knees cannot be brought within $2^1/2$ inches of the floor, this is a risk factor for back pain.

2. As seen in figure (4-b), this is a simple way to measure progress in this exercise, if the range of motion of both legs is similar.

3. As seen in figure (4-c), if one groin stretches only to a definite firm stopping point while the other groin shows a more progressive gradual stretching process, this is considered a risk factor for back pain and often an indication of psoas tendon shortening.

4. As seen in figure (4-d), if the difference between knees is measured to be more than 1 inch further off the floor, this is considered a risk factor for back pain on that side.

5. As seen in figure (4-d), if the individual is unable to comfortably place one leg on the floor and maintain balance in this position, this is also considered a risk factor.

5. Sitting Knee to Cross Chest – Pyriformis stretch

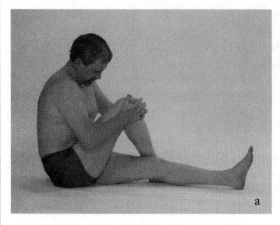 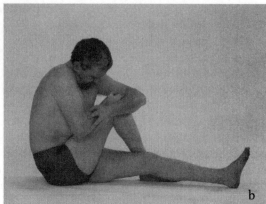

a. Sitting position with the right foot on the other side of the opposite leg.
b. Pull right knee toward the left shoulder. Repeat for opposite side.

Notes: This stretch is difficult to measure accurately.

Risk Factors:
1. Any noticeable tightness or difference in range of motion.
2. Any difference in tenderness of the stretch response.

6. KNEELING WIDE STANCE PELVIS TO FLOOR – ILIOPSOAS STRETCH

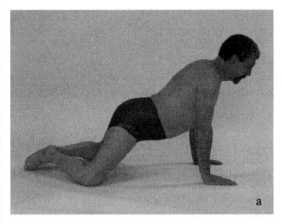 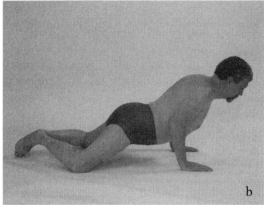

a. Kneeling position with knees at least shoulder width apart or preferably as wide as possible.
b. Slowly attempt to place the pelvis area of the body to the floor. Arch or extend the back forward. The soles of the feet should be touching each other. If this is not a comfortable position, leave the feet spread apart. However, the feet must be the same distance apart and pointed in a precisely symmetrical fashion.

Notes: This is a difficult stretching exercise to measure accurately.

Risk factors:
1. The major stretch area is in the groin. If you feel the pull in one groin area more than the other does, this constitutes a risk factor.
2. If the pull in the groin is symmetrical but one foot has to be moved to achieve this sensation, this also constitutes a risk factor.

7. KNEELING ELBOWS BACK TO FLOOR – QUADRICEPS STRETCH

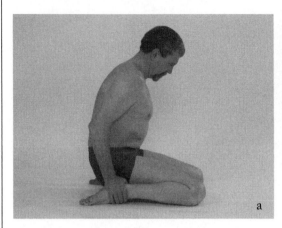 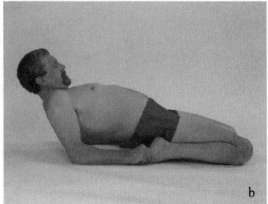

a. In the kneeling position, slowly lean backwards. Be sure to support the body weight with both arms. Feet should be at least pelvis width apart and pointed backwards or at a 45-degree angle. Make certain the feet are not pointed outwards at a 90-degree angle. This can put extreme stress on the inner aspect of the knees.

b. Support yourself with both arms until nearly the full range of motion has been obtained. When the buttocks can be placed on the floor, carefully lower the weight of the body to one elbow. If comfortable, lower the weight to the second elbow.

Notes:
1. Ideally this exercise should be done with a spotter to help you back up should the stretch on the quadriceps become too great.
2. Some individuals can then lower the back onto the floor. Due to the complexity, this position is not recommended. A spotter is definitely required to attain this position for safety reasons.
3. There should be no significant stress on either the knees or ankles.

Risk factors:
1. A minor risk factor exists if the stretch on the front of one thigh is greater than on the front of the other thigh.

8. PRONE TWISTING CRAWL – LUMBAR ROTATOR MUSCLES

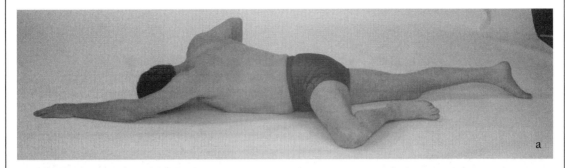

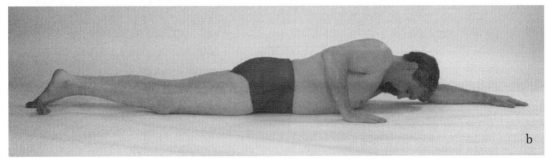

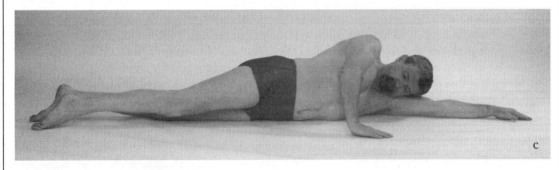

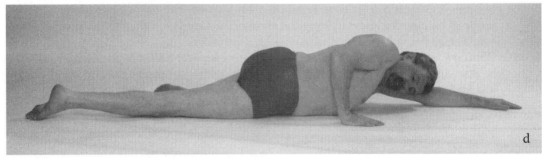

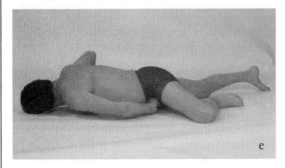

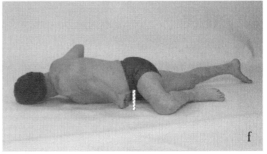

8. PRONE TWISTING CRAWL – LUMBAR ROTATOR MUSCLES (CONTINUED)

a. In the prone position, extend the left arm fully above the head and bring the left leg to a 90 degree position as if to crawl. As seen from the left.

b. Due to the complexity of the stretch, it is broken down into various steps. First start this complex exercise in the prone position by extending the left arm fully above the head.

c. With the right arm in a push up position, push the right side of the body to a 45 degree roll.

d. Return to neutral and bring the left leg to a 90 degree angle and slowly attempt the roll. This puts a tremendous amount of twisting motion to the low back.

e-f. Measure the height of the left groin from the floor.

Notes:

1. If the back is tight, this motion will cause the low back to pop. Sometimes up to 3 separate pops at 3 levels of the low back can be both felt and heard. This popping sensation should disappear after the first 2 weeks of exercise. If it does not disappear, this stretch should be discontinued. The goal is not to pop the back but to loosen the lumbar muscles so the back doesn't pop.

2. The stretch should be felt primarily in the mid-line of the low back just above the pelvis level.

3. The stretch should also be felt in the groin area of the left side. Often the stretching sensation will feel the same. However, the distance the groin is to the floor can be significantly different. This distance can be measured in two different ways. First a level and tape measure can measure the height of the pelvis from the floor. A second way is to measure with the hand the height of the groin off the floor (see figure e. and f.).

4. Although difficult to measure, it is important to determine if the height of pelvis off the floor is more than 1/2 inch higher than the other side. This measurement does not need to be repeated on a regular basis as it seldom changes significantly. This is presumed to be largely due to tendon shortening.

5. Due to the fragility of these muscles do not exceed mild stretch or do only the warm up and avoid the Opti-stretch phase.

Risk factors:

1. If the height of the groin off the floor has more than a 1/2 inch different between sides, this is a very important risk factor to determine. In this situation, the muscles of the buttocks are first contracted in order to bring the groin of the bent leg as close to the floor as possible. Then a twisting motion of the low back is performed.

2. If the low back continues to pop on a regular basis for over a month, the exercise should be discontinued. The rationale is that popping of joints over prolonged periods of time can lead to hypertrophy of the joint capsule in certain joints.

9. SITTING CHEERLEADER – NOSE TO KNEE
10. SITTING CHEERLEADER – ELBOW TO ANKLE
11. SITTING CHEERLEADER – HIP TO CROSS KNEE

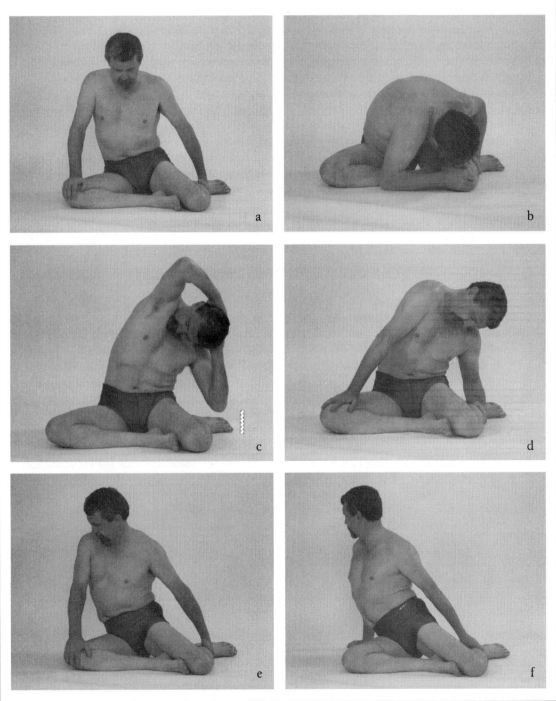

Sitting Cheerleader (CONTINUED)

a. The cheerleader pose is in the sitting position with the right leg bent at a 90 degree angle and the left leg bent outwards with extension backwards. There are 3 separate stretching exercises, which are performed on both the left and right sides.

b. The "Nose to Knee" exercise is to slowly attempt to touch the nose to the left knee. The stretch is felt in the left front area of the thigh near the left hip. Measure the distance.

c. The "Elbow to Ankle" exercise is to place the hands behind the head and slowly attempt to touch the left elbow to the left ankle. This allows determination of the general plane of motion. Measure the distance between the elbow and ankle.

d. With the right hand on the right knee and the left hand on the left calf, attempt to touch the left ankle with the forearm. The stretch is felt in the left hip and lateral thigh. This position is used as the stretching exercise.

e. The "Hip to Cross Knee" exercise is started with the left hand grabbing the left ankle. The right hand is on the right knee.

f. Slowly attempt to bring the left hip forward and toward the right knee while holding the left ankle. The stretch is felt in the left groin area. For balance, the right hand can be placed on the floor.

Notes: Frequently the stretch is felt in the inner aspect of the left knee in both the "Elbow to Ankle" and the "Nose to Knee" exercise stretches. Care should be taken not to overly stretch the knee area.

Risk factors:

1. Frequently, it is even difficult to sit maintaining normal balance on one side versus the other in the normal cheerleader pose. This is a risk factor for the tighter side.

2. In either the "Elbow to Ankle" or the "Nose to Knee" exercise stretches, if the stretch exceeds 1 inch on the left side compared with the right side, the tighter side is considered to have a risk factor.

3. In the "Hip to Cross Knee" stretching exercise, if any sensation of extra tightness compared with the other side is found, this again is a risk factor for the tighter groin area.

12. KNEELING NARROW STANCE PELVIS TO FLOOR – (COBRA)

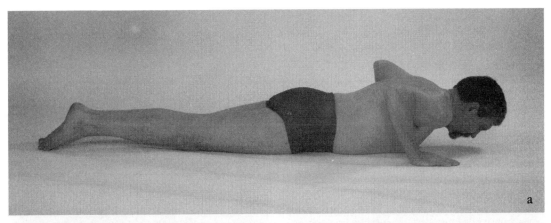

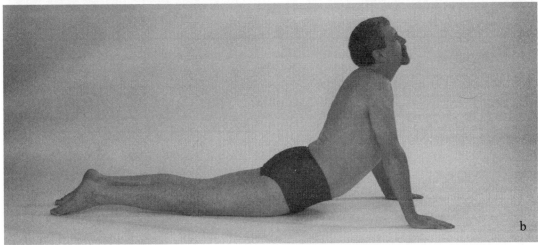

a. Start in the prone position.
b. From the prone position, slowly elevate the upper body leaving the pelvis on the floor. This should put a stretch on the low back.

Notes: This position is extremely gravity dependent on the low back and should be done very carefully.

Risk factors:
    1. The stretch is felt primarily in the low back, but also in the groin areas. If a stretch can be felt more in one groin than the other, this is considered a risk factor.
    2. If it can be felt on one side of the lower back more than the other, this also is a risk factor.

13. Rhomboid Pull – Greater and Less Rhomboid Muscle Exercise

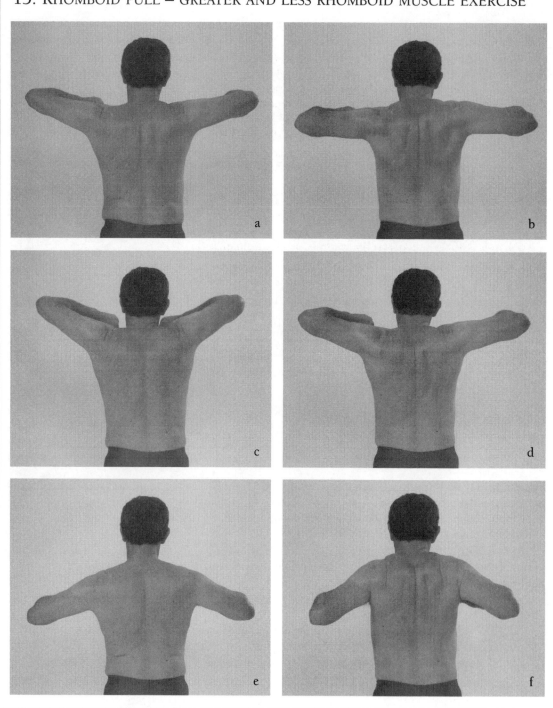

13. RHOMBOID PULL (CONTINUED)

a-b. In either the standing or kneeling position, place the arms out level and horizontal. Bend the elbows so the hands are close to the chest. Pull the elbows toward the back as if to touch the elbows together. The forearms should be pointing in a downward direction. The hands should be clenched.

c-d. Place the elbows 2 inches above level and repeat the process.

e-f. Place the elbows 2 inches below level and repeat the process.

Notes: The stretch should be felt in the front of the shoulders on each side. However, the important sensation is the tightening sensation between the shoulder blades.

Risk factors:

1. If the pull and muscle tightness or tenderness can be felt more on the right or left of midline in the shoulder blade area, the tighter side has the risk factor for a rhomboid chronic injured muscle. The goal is to be able to pull very slowly to full strength and have the tension felt in-between the shoulder blades feel equal.

14. Finger Touch – rhomboid, trapezius and shoulder rotators

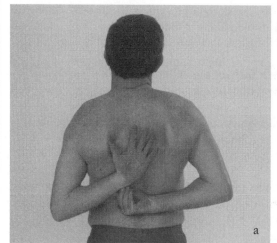

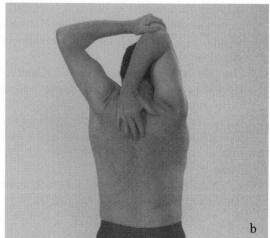

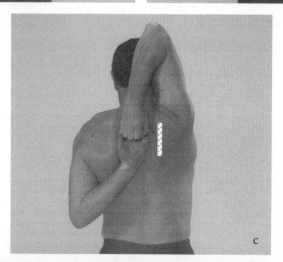

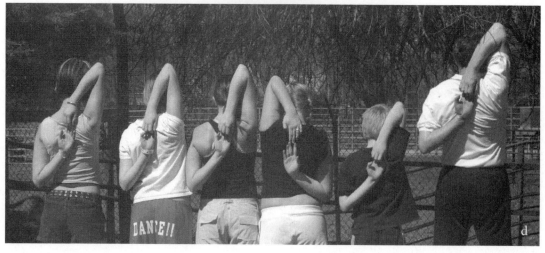

14. FINGER TOUCH (CONTINUED)

a. In either the kneeling or standing position reach the left hand behind the back and attempt to touch the lower scapular area. Repeat on the other side.

b. Next attempt to reach over the shoulder with the right hand and touch the upper scapular area. Repeat on the other side.

c. Then attempt to touch the fingers. Fingers should be overlapped but not grabbed for measuring the "Finger Touch". Following measurement, the fingers can be grabbed to increase the stretch on the shoulders.

d. This stretching exercise is usually quite easy for younger children. An optimum "Finger Touch" is where the fingers can overlap to nearly touch the palm of the hands. When the fingers are grabbed, they allow for optimum range of motion of the shoulders.

Notes: Reaching the hand behind the back to the lower scapular area puts a significant strain on the same side anterior joint capsule of the shoulder and rotator cuff. Proceed very slowly and be especially careful not to strain the anterior shoulder area.

Risk factors:

1. A 1-inch difference measured between the fingertips comparing the two sides is a risk factor. Then measure the absolute height of each arm. Determine which is the tighter shoulder. The tighter shoulder is a risk factor for upper back and neck pain on that particular side.

2. If the fingertip touch is fairly symmetrical on both sides but the distance between fingertips exceeds 2 inches, this should also be considered a relative risk factor.

15. CHIN TO SHOULDER

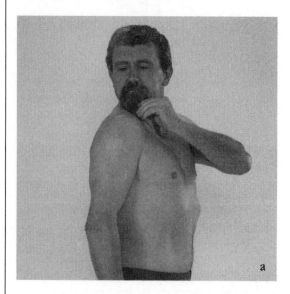

a.   Place the left hand on the chin and gently push the chin so it is pointing at a 90-degree angle. The tip of the chin should be pointing directly toward the center of the right shoulder.

Note:
1.   The neck is extremely sensitive to stretching exercises. Be sure to proceed extra slowly and carefully to avoid injury.
2.   Repeat the process on the opposite side.

Risk factors:
1.   If the range of motion is ½ inch less on one side compared to the other side, this is a risk factor for neck pain on the side demonstrating the tighter muscle.
2.   When the chin is placed on the right shoulder, the stretch is often felt on both sides of the neck. However, the stretch should primarily be felt on the opposite side (left side). If the primary stretch is felt on the same side (right side in this case), this is considered a risk factor.

16. CHIN BACKWARDS

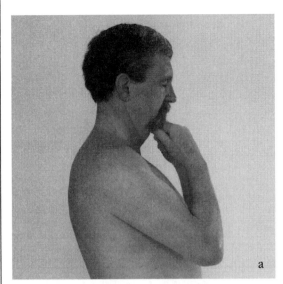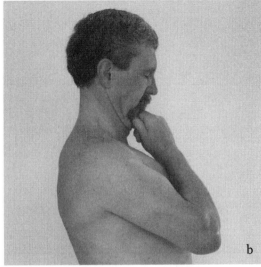

a.   This is a difficult stretch to perform correctly. In the standing position, place the dominant hand on the chin. Next place the other hand over the dominant hand. Close the mouth firmly for support but do not clench the teeth. Place the head in a slightly forward position.

b.   Slowly apply backward pressure to the chin while exhaling. The stretch should be felt in the neck at the base of the skull.

Notes: It may be necessary to try various levels of head tilt to find the maximum level of stretch at the back of the neck. Be particularly careful not to make the jaw area sore.

Risk factors:
1.   If one side of the base of the skull feels tighter than the other, this is considered a risk factor.

17. EAR TO SHOULDER
18. STRAIGHT ARM EAR TO SHOULDER

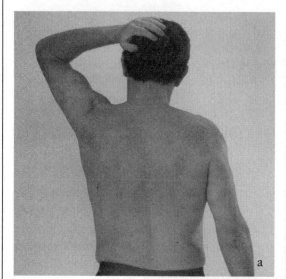 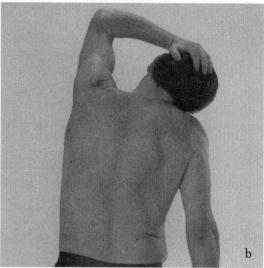

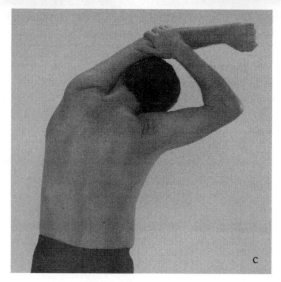

a. In either the standing or sitting position, allow the head to tilt sideways touching the right ear towards the right shoulder. Do not elevate the shoulder.

b. Very gently provide a slight amount of stretch with either hand. Be careful! The neck can be easily strained in this position.

c. A safer way to stretch the neck laterally and provide an excellent shoulder stretch is to bring the left straight arm to the ear. With the right arm, provide the force to bring the right ear to the right shoulder.

Notes: This is one of the more sensitive stretches. It must be performed slowly and carefully to avoid any neck strain.

Risk factors:
1. If the one ear is further away from the shoulder compared with the other ear, this is a risk factor for the opposite side of the neck.
2. If one side of the neck feels tighter, this is also a risk factor.

19. CHIN TO CHEST

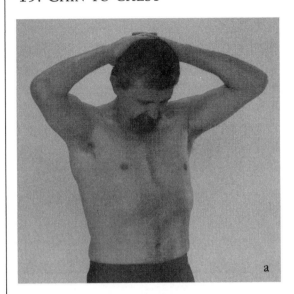

a.   Place the hands behind the head and gently lower the chin toward the chest.

Notes: This is usually an easy stretch for most individuals.

Risk factors:
1.   If the chin does not come within one inch of the chest, this is a risk factor.
2.   If tightness is felt in back of the neck on one side more significantly than the other, this is a risk factor.

20. EAR TO AXILLA (ARMPIT)

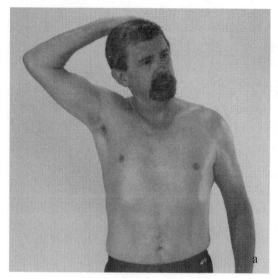 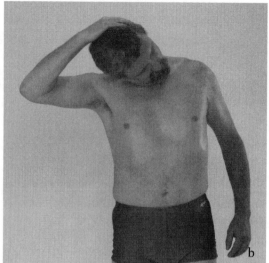

a. In the standing or sitting position, turn the head to the left by approximately 45 degrees. The head should still be in an upright position.
b. Using the right hand or both hands, gently pull the head so the right ear is moving in the direction of the right armpit (axilla).

Notes: This is a very sensitive stretch. It must be performed in a very slow and careful manner so as to avoid injury.

Risk Factors:
1. This stretch is difficult to measure. However, if one side feels tighter than the other, this is considered a risk factor.

ASSESSMENT OF SCREENING TESTS

■ ■ ■

The Opti-stretch Beginning and Intermediate Screening Tests evaluate for risk factors. Determination that certain anatomical risk factors for recurrent back pain actually existed was the second most important discovery in Opti-stretch research. The most important discovery was that risk factors could be corrected in order to regain a healthy back.

In my 23-year battle with recurrent back strain, I had input from the very best physicians in America. However, I intuitively knew that there had to be something that was different with me compared with the majority of my friends. With increasing age and traveling to multiple geographic regions of the USA and other countries, I started encountering a handful of friends with the same desire for high activity levels who had exactly the same recurrent back strain pattern that I did. They too, after each back strain were told to go home, rest, gradually increase activity levels, and their backs would get better. For a time, yes, this would indeed occur. However, inevitably something would come along, to restrain that precise area of their backs. Like me, they simply lived with the problem. Many were MDs, who had reverted to seeing alternative medicine physicians for this recurrent medical problem.

Risk factors are anatomical differences that an individual can actually see for themselves. Because of the very precise reproducibility of these differences and the ability to accurately measure them, these anatomical parameters can be followed and correlated with having a healthy back or not. Finally, I could actually see something different in me compared with those having healthy backs. This allowed me to correct the problem.

Presented in this book are only the simplified basics of risk factor assessment. Each "recurrent back pain syndrome" has a very characteristic pattern of several groups of muscles with ACIMs, which can then exhibit varying degrees of chronic injury spasm. Moreover, each syndrome has multiple normal variants. An entire book could be devoted to this one subject alone. This is in part due to the complexity of anatomical variations in the various human races. Currently, there are 18 different genetic anatomical variations of just the psoas muscle complex, which incidentally consists of only 3 muscles. It is currently believed that the anatomical variations do not cause the back pain. However, should an injury occur, certain anatomical variations are more susceptible to forming "recurrent back strain syndromes". (See Section II – Scientific Considerations #14. The Psoas Muscle.)

As mentioned previously, just because certain risk factors are present does not mean you will have back pain. The ability to comfortably perform certain of the Advanced

Program stretches (i.e., Standing Squat), seems to allow a great deal of protection from developing the initial significant low back strain.

An Opti-stretch Therapeutic Program should be strongly considered if any of the following could be demonstrated during the screening exams:

1. risk factors (as described for each individual exercise)
2. unequal range of motion – (asymmetry)
3. very limited range of motion

For the 20% of the population with no risk factors, no asymmetry and good range of motion, these fortunate individuals need to simply record their range of motion. This information could be extremely valuable if a severe accident or injury were to occur. These individuals should consider repeating the screening test periodically. This can be either every 6 months or annually.

Remember that Opti-stretch is designed for <u>primary</u> chronically injured muscles (ACIMs). However, it may be helpful in certain forms of <u>secondary</u> chronically injured muscles. **It was not designed for treating acute injuries or acute reinjuries**. In the early stages of acute injury, the inflammatory stage can even be prolonged with Opti-stretch. Chronically injured muscles and mild acute injuries can often feel very similar. If you are having muscle pain or even mild discomfort at rest, there may be an acute injury process going on. Once you have learned the Opti-stretch technique, it can be helpful in acute injury situations after the muscle has <u>healed</u> for a specific period of time (roughly 2 days). Discussion of time periods for various strains is found in Step #2 of the Opti-stretch Challenge and in the Scientific Considerations section.

Something must happen to initially cause the first significant injury. The majority of the time this is most commonly due to lifting a heavy object. In acute reinjury, often very subtle forces can cause the reinjury. Take for example a mild acute reinjury to the muscle. Most commonly, there is a sensation of a pulled muscle or pain at the time of injury. However, quite often, the pain will not occur until you wake up the following morning. This represents two different severity's of acute injury. Different severity's of injury take different times to heal. As a general rule of thumb, you should be at least 2 months out from any acute injury before performing the screening tests or learning the Opti-stretch technique, <u>even with mild injuries</u>. Also, a medical doctor should reevaluate any pain lasting more than 2 months and not following a normal healing pattern. However, once you have initially learned the program this type of mild injury can usually receive benefit from gentle Opti-stretch stretching exercise after a couple of days rest.

STEP #2 OF THE OPTI-STRETCH CHALLENGE IS THE THERAPEUTIC TECHNIQUE APPLIED TO THE BEGINNING AND INTERMEDIATE PROGRAMS

■ ■ ■

In Step #2 you will learn the stretching technique that Opti-stretch has found to be most helpful in returning tight and tender muscles (ACIMs) to normally toned muscles.

There are a couple of important topics that need to be covered. Stretching properly is complex. First, the terminology often has different meanings to different people. The body has several different types of stretch receptors that serve different functions. Stretching is simply applying an increasing force to a joint or joints to put stress on the muscle to increase the range of motion. If the same force is applied rapidly to a tendon the muscle will reflexively contract (like a doctor hitting your knee with a reflex hammer). This is a protective reflex. Muscles themselves possess several different types of stretch receptors. The most familiar ones are the stretch receptors that warn when the muscle is being "stretched", to a specific range of motion. If this gradually increasing force continues to be applied, the sensation of stretch changes to a sensation of discomfort. The levels of discomfort can be referred to as mild, moderate, and severe. If the stretching force continues to gradually increase, the severe discomfort sensation progresses to a pain sensation. At the pain threshold level, the muscle will usually experience some type of microscopic injury.

Muscles have two opposite functions. One is to contract and <u>move</u> a joint through a range of motion. The other function is to spasm and <u>immobilize</u> a joint. This spasm is an important part of the healing process. The muscle gradually relaxes the spasm over days to weeks, depending on the extent of injury. The muscle can spasm in response to various types of pain stimulus from surrounding structures. This can be due to muscle tissue injury, injury to the surrounding connective tissue (myofascia), or injury of a tendon, bone or joint. Any of these injuries will result in spasm and an acute injured muscle. During the first few days of a severe injury, there are injury stretch receptors that protect the muscle and joint structures. Early injury stretch receptors can detect very little of any type of stretch sensation. Instead, even slight movement will transition directly to the pain state. As the muscle heals, a warning level of discomfort will develop before the level of pain is reached. As the muscle more fully heals, the level of a stretch sensation then reoccurs.

Stretching exercises can be used as a tool in several specific functions. The Opti-stretch Therapeutic Technique utilizes the first three of these four functions. The specific functions of stretching exercises are as follows:

1. Detection of both acute and chronic injuries. (Risk factors can then be detected in the chronic injury state, which most commonly involve asymptomatic chronic muscle injuries (ACIMs) or tendon shortening.)
2. Warming up the muscles (mild intensity only).
3. Therapeutically stretching the muscles so over time the range of motion of the muscle will be improved. (The goal is to optimally stretch the muscle and restore proper tone, so that the stretch receptor is lengthened allowing further range of motion for a given intensity of force delivered to the muscle.)
   3.1 Documentation that you have achieved at least two inches of increased stretch (stretch receptor lengthening.)
4. Cooling Down Muscles after a hard workout to prevent stiffness and soreness.

A Brief Overview of the Therapeutic Technique for Stretch Receptor Lengthening
(used for Beginning and Intermediate Programs).

Therapeutically stretching the muscles requires certain **special techniques**:

1. Breathing Technique (Incremental exhaling during stretch and inhaling during relaxation of the stretch. Forced exhalation used in The Therapeutic Phase).
2. Incremental Movement Technique (Uses 3 progressive incremental stretches of approximately 1/4 inch with only partial relaxation after each incremental stretch).
3. Intensity of Force Technique as determined by different levels of discomfort. A properly toned muscle will have 4 sensations of stretch discomfort before the level of pain is reached (see Table 1, page 83 and Graph 1, page 88).
   3.1 Determination of the "first sensation of stretch" (whenever any sensation of stretch occurs in any area of the body). Distance stretched from the "first sensation of stretch" to the next noticeable change in discomfort "second sensation of stretch" is the **mild discomfort** stretch range.
   3.2 Distance stretched from the "second sensation of stretch" to the "third sensation of stretch" is the **moderate discomfort** stretch range.
   3.3 Distance stretched from the "third sensation of stretch" to the "fourth sensation of stretch" is the **moderately-severe discomfort** stretch range.
   3.4 Distance stretched from the "fourth sensation of stretch" to the "first sensation of pain" is the **severe discomfort** stretch range. This stretch range is for learning purposes only! Just 3 specific stretching exercises are suitable for this intensity level.

The "fifth sensation of stretch" starts the "mild pain" range. This intensity of stretch level should never be reached, otherwise injury will likely occur.

THE INCREMENTAL BREATHING TECHNIQUE

The following two techniques for breathing and movement are necessary in order to have optimum success. Unless these two concepts are fully understood, chances are high that either an injury will occur or the benefits you are seeking will take a long time in coming.

The breathing technique may sound simple but is very important. There appears to be normal reflex mechanisms in the body that allow muscles to relax while exhaling. There are also mechanical factors that allow the core muscles of the lower and upper back to stretch slightly further after forced exhalation.

First pronounce the letter "O". Keep the mouth in the same position. Next, practice exhaling so a slight blowing sound of air can be heard both by you and another person, if they were standing beside you. Approximately one third of the lung volume should be expelled each time you think to yourself the numbers: one, two, three. The cadence is one number every 1 to 1½ seconds. This will exhale most of the air from the lungs. Next, think of the word "and". While saying "and" you inhale for 2 to 3 seconds. The rate should be relaxing, slow and rhythmical. It does take a little practice to judge the amount of air to both exhale and inhale so that you neither get short of breath nor hyperventilate.

INCREMENTAL MOVEMENT TECHNIQUE

The cadence is "1-2-3-and". Start by finding the point of the "first sensation of stretch". Very slowly and gently stretch ¼ inch or less for each of the three numbers. Approximately ½ the distance across the nail bed is the maximum amount of a slow gentle stretching movement that you will want to make while thinking each number. This means ¾ inch is accomplished in 3 smooth and gentle movements. During the "and" segment, the stretch is relaxed by one half inch while breathing in. Therefore, for each cadence, the total distance progressed into the stretch is only ¼ inch.

OPTI-STRETCH STRETCHING SEQUENCE

Properly stretching a muscle to achieve stretch receptor lengthening is best achieved using an "Opti-stretch Stretching Sequence". This is composed of a detection phase, a warm-up phase and a therapeutic phase. Each is performed somewhat differently. Located in Graph 3, page 177, is a diagrammatic presentation of the following description.

The <u>detection phase</u> (Check and Stretch) is used to determine if there are any minor acute injuries to the muscles. In the comfortable ready position, the stretching exercise is slowly performed only to the level of the "first sensation of stretch" (Check). This is the first part of the <u>detection phase</u>. Opti-stretch research has demonstrated that this point is reached at a very similar location of stretch for many groups of individuals and for different conditions of the muscle tissue. The distance into the stretch is easily memorized. If you detect this distance to have shortened or is noticeably more uncomfortable than previously, the likelihood of an acute injury is high (stop stretching for at least two days to allow time for the muscle to start healing). Gently detect the "first sensation of stretch" three times and then return to the ready position. Repeat the process a second time. This should take only 6 to 12 seconds.

The second part of the <u>detection phase</u> is the "stretch". Go to the "first sensation of stretch". This is by definition the start of mild discomfort stretch. The stretch is slowly and cautiously continued to where there is any noticeable change in this mild sensation of stretch. This point is a "second sensation of stretch". This is depicted diagrammatically in **Graph 1** – <u>Muscle Stretch to Pain Transition</u>, page 88. Unless there is an acute injury, this transition point is the start of moderate discomfort stretch. For certain sized muscles and also poorly toned muscle this stretch distance could be less than 2 inches. In a optimally toned muscle it could be 6 or 8 inches. There are 4 of these easily recognizable transition points before the onset of mild pain in any large muscle that is healthy. It is around this second transition point (transition from mild to moderate discomfort) that you will perform the warm up phase and the therapeutic phase. After months in the program, other transition points can safely be worked at.

The <u>warm-up phase</u> is used to properly warm up the muscles so that you are able to proceed with the therapeutic phase. A slight modification of the classic incremental movement technique is used. At an intensity force level causing mild discomfort, the incremental movements are held for 1 second with gentle exhalation (<u>Table 1</u> – <u>Therapeutic Intensity Levels for Stretching</u>, page 83). During "and" the intensity of force is partially released and a breath is inhaled. The cadence is (5-4-3-2-1-"and"). This process allows for slight increases in range of motion while using the exact same intensity level of mild discomfort. This cadence is repeated two more times.

The <u>Opti-stretch Therapeutic Phase</u> uses Opti-stretch incremental breathing technique, incremental movement technique and a maximum forced exhalation. Using the <u>incremental breathing</u> and <u>incremental movement</u> technique, explained on the previous page, the cadence is (1-2-3-"and"). This is referred to as a <u>subset</u>. Initially, 3 Opti-stretch subsets are performed and then followed by a forced exhalation. This is referred to as the Opti-stretch Therapeutic phase.

A <u>set</u> consists of a Detection Phase, a Warm Up Phase and two Opti-stretch Therapeutic Phases. A total of 3 sets (separated by 1-minute rests) are performed for each exercise during the daily exercise routine. [(Graph 3) in the Appendix, page 177]

Following 2 months of daily Opti-stretch, a third Opti-stretch Therapeutic Phase can be added to the set and is then referred to as an <u>intermediate set</u>.

During the incremental exhalation, slow cautious range of motion increases are performed. A predetermined intensity level is chosen before an Opti-stretch Therapeutic Phase is attempted. Over weeks and months of continued daily exercise, the muscles gradually become more toned and range of motion is optimized for the given body type.

Of special note, the <u>forced exhalation</u> is performed after the third Opti-stretch subset. The chest is contracted to slowly but forcefully exhale the last residual lung volume. The forceful exhalation often allows 1 full inch of increased range of motion without any further increase in the intensity of discomfort level. **Do not exceed 1 inch**, even if you think you safely can. Serious strain injuries have occurred by exceeding this 1-inch limit (especially when the muscles have become more toned). This is the end of the Opti-stretch therapeutic phase (3 subsets and a forced exhalation). The stretch is then released to the intensity level of discomfort where you started into that Opti-stretch phase. The therapeutic phase is repeated a second time in order to complete one set. [(Graph 3) in Appendix, page 177]

<u>Warning.</u> Complex anatomical, physiological and even psychological forces are combined during the forced exhalation part of the Opti-stretch Therapeutic Phase. While very effective and helpful in daily increases in range of motion, once the muscles have become toned, several individuals have reported comfortable 3 to 6 inch gains in range of motion during the forced exhalation. This excess distance can be **<u>very dangerous</u>**. A sudden tearing of the muscle covering called the myofascia can occur without any warning. This can cause a severe muscle strain. These individuals reported no sensation of discomfort; they simply heard a "pop". Shortly thereafter, the muscle became extremely painful and had been seriously strained. Remember not to exceed the recommended 1 inch of extra stretch during forced exhalation. For this and several other reasons, **<u>do not use Opti-stretch techniques on any other stretching exercises except those demonstrated in this book!</u>**

Follow the sequence of the stretches shown in the book. The most important exercises are shown first. This allows the most important exercises to be completed if there happens to be a time constraint that particular day. Furthermore, during the one minute rests between exercise sets, muscles on the opposite side of the body can then be stretched. For those exercises that stretch both sides of the body at the same time, go to the next exercise, which usually starts in a similar position (i.e., kneeling). After a week or two of learning the technique, start with the tighter side first. A total of 3 sets are performed on the tighter side, and 2 sets on the more flexible side. This will help correct the asymmetry more smoothly. If more than an inch of stretch receptor lengthening occurs on the more flexible side without an increase in the tighter side, you may have to cut even more sets from the more flexible side. **Do not** promote the asymmetry by more than 2 additional inches from your initial screening test without adjusting your program. (see Table 4, page 175).

Following 2 months of working in the "second sensation of stretch" (transition between mild and moderate discomfort) the second Opti-stretch set can be performed further into the moderate discomfort level. No more than two sets should be performed at any predetermined higher intensity level. The muscles become fatigued and the chance of injury is higher. This is one instance where "more is not better".

For the first 2 to 8 weeks of practicing Opti-stretch stretching exercises, do not go any further than the intensity level of a mild discomfort and the beginning of moderate discomfort. If you seem comfortable with these levels and start to see results, stay at that level. However, if you want to try a more aggressive, efficacious, and slightly more risky level from an injury standpoint, the <u>Optimum Opti-stretch intensity level</u> is presented. Even for "extreme" individuals and those who push the envelope on any physical activity they engage in, the following is the <u>most intense level</u> that should be tried.

The safest way to start learning about this maximum Opti-stretch intensity level is by practicing stretching the fingers. Here you can learn with tendon and joint stretch receptors that are more sensitive than core muscle stretch receptors. Extend all 4 fingers of the left hand backward with the right hand. This is performed both slowly and gently until you feel a mild stretch. Release the stretch and move both hands to see if there is a sensation of continued stretching on any finger. Wait at least one minute. If there is no sensation of a continuing sensation of stretch after the stretch has been released (residual stretch), repeat the process to what you think a moderate discomfort stretch level might be.

If no level of residual stretch has been obtained, repeat the above sequence on the same 4 fingers increasing the stretch slightly by only 1/16th of an inch past your level of moderate discomfort. Continue noting the difference in the sensation between the mild, moderate, and the new moderately-severe discomfort level. Eventually, there will be a point where a sensation of residual stretch occurs for less than 15 to 60 seconds. This is, by definition, the <u>severe discomfort</u> level. The level of stretch just prior to this and following your moderate discomfort level is by definition the moderately-severe discomfort range. This sensation of moderately-severe discomfort should be memorized. It is the most effective intensity range that you can safely work in and still avoid overstretching injuries. You <u>never</u> want to enter the intensity level of mild "pain" (which is a residual sensation of stretch that lasts from 1 to 5 minutes). Any residual sensation of stretch lasting more than 5 minutes is likely due to a strain injury. Over the next 2 to 8 hours, this can result in very painful spasm of the muscle. (See Table 1, page 83).

Practice this technique only on the (Figure Four), the (Butterfly) or "Supine Straight Knee to Nose" stretching exercises. <u>Less</u> than this level of intensity must be used on all of the other stretching exercises. **<u>Remember</u>!! You have stretched too far if:**

1. <u>**Any sensation of residual stretch is felt.**</u> **If the residual discomfort lasts for more than five minutes, consider this to be an acute injury and wait two days before resuming the stretching exercises.**

2. <u>Any stiffness or soreness occurs the following day</u>.
3. **In repeating a stretch, the level of moderate discomfort is reached <u>noticeably sooner</u> than from a prior stretch.**

Most people see a definite improvement in the stretching distance (stretch receptor lengthening) in 2 to 3 months. If no improvement is noted, you may need to consult with a qualified instructor to determine if there might be something in your technique that could be improved. It may take up to 6 months to achieve your own specific goals, depending on your preexisting muscle tone and your age.

<u>The following is a very important point to remember!</u>

The above Opti-stretch technique is based solely on sensation of the muscles and not by achieving the same distance of stretch as you did the day before. The muscles and their stretch receptors are a very dynamic system. If there is a little bit of extra lactic acid build up from the prior days' activities, if you are a little run down, stressed, or if a cold is coming on, you may not be able to reach the same level of stretch as you did the day before. If you then try to obtain the same range or a little further than the day before, you will eventually injure a muscle.

The best way to avoid this is to perform the Opti-stretch Technique with the eyes closed or partially closed. If you are focusing on reaching a certain distance of stretching you are <u>not</u> fully concentrating on what the muscles are telling you. Therefore, you will eventually strain a muscle with stretching exercises. This is even more important the older you are. Use the <u>measured distances</u> only as a guide to weekly or monthly progress.

VARIATIONS IN STEP # 2

Step #2 or the Opti-stretch Therapeutic Technique may be accomplished in different ways. Some people find that just trying to get into the basic starting position for certain exercises in the Intermediate Therapeutic Program is difficult. For this reason a <u>Beginning Program </u>has been constructed. After achieving good range of motion on these stretching exercises, return to the Intermediate stretches.

For time constraints, the Low Back exercises (Screening Exercises 1-12) in the Intermediate Screening Program should be mastered first during the first couple of weeks. Then start incorporating the Upper Back and Neck exercises (especially if this is where the areas of recurrent pain are located). The goal is to both obtain equal movement on each side of the body and obtain as close to the "gold standard" as possible.

If you have only neck pain, carefully test for asymmetry of the lower and upper back. If there is asymmetry, the neck muscles are difficult to fully rehabilitate if the lower and upper back asymmetry is not corrected first. If there is a time constraint, you are better off to first correct the lower back, then the upper back and then the neck.

If you have a 20-minute daily time constraint, you may have to then tailor your Therapeutic Program to your own particular needs. Always work first on the low back. My particular routine is as follows: Intermediate Screening Exercises 1-14, and then starting to gradually add in Advanced Exercises 3 and 8. Advanced Exercises 4 and 7 are then periodically worked on. On the weekends or 2 to 3 days a week spend some time on the Upper Back and Neck exercises. After 2 to 4 months of the Low Back stretching exercises, you will find the goals on Upper Back and Neck exercises will be achieved both faster and easier.

A synopsis of the daily exercise routine is provided in the Appendix, on the Beginning and Intermediate Worksheets.

NOTE:
The "Therapeutic Technique" applied to the
"Intermediate Program" is often referred to as the
"Intermediate Therapeutic Program".

NOTES

_____

_____

_____

_____

_____

_____

_____

_____

TABLE 1. – THERAPEUTIC INTENSITY LEVELS FOR STRETCHING

Sensation level	Micro-stretch level	Sensation after relaxing the stretch	Actions
First Sensation of Stretch	25 % MAX	None	Continue stretching
Mild Discomfort	50% MAX	None	Continue stretching
Moderate Discomfort	80% MAX	None	A sufficient ending point.
Moderately-severe Discomfort	100% MAX	None	Maximum ending point.
Severe Discomfort		Sensation of continued stretch for < 1 minute	Be aware that there could be an injury. Continue stretching cautiously.
Mild Pain		Sensation of continued stretch for 1-5 minutes	Stop stretching for 2 days
Moderate Pain		Sensation of continued stretch for > 5 minutes	Stop stretching and only very conservative activities for the next 6-8 hours. If pain progresses to a severe level, seek medical attention. Stop stretching for at least 5-7 days to allow healing.

Certain basic concepts and principles need to be understood to insure optimum results and prevent injury. In order to achieve this, specific definitions to the sometimes-confusing terminology of back pain are provided below.

CLASSIFICATIONS OF BACK PAIN VS. RECURRENT BACK STRAIN

In order to understand "recurrent back strain", it is important to see how it compares to all types of back pain. Because "recurrent back strain" is new to many, a description of the criteria used to determine various types of injury are presented. Remember, only a doctor can determine for sure that you have a muscle strain and not something more serious.

BACK PAIN

Back pain is a commonly misunderstood term. Back pain is composed of several different types.

20% of the population statistically have <u>never had any back pain</u>. Interviewing and studying the range of motion of this group of individuals was invaluable in formulating many of the goals and concepts of Opti-stretch.

80% – Have had at least one episode of significant back pain.

- 15% – Malignant (occurring in severe form and commonly referred to as pathologic). Spine fractures, herniated discs, infection, tumor, etc. There are approximately 25 to 30 different pathologic disease processes, each that have a very specific form of therapy. Usually arthritic and chronic persistent back pain problems are in this group.

- 85% – Benign. Benign back pain is also sometimes referred to as common back pain. It is usually diagnosed as a muscle strain or fascial (soft tissue and ligament strain) which is most commonly referred to as myofascial strain. The majority of time it is associated with lifting a heavy object or twisting while lifting. It is a clinical diagnosis and no x-rays or blood tests can more specifically diagnose the muscle or tissue involved. Commonly the only form of therapy is rest and reassurance it will get better on its own.

- >50% – Heal fine and do not reoccur.
- ? % – A significantly large number of these individuals religiously avoid the same level of activity that caused the initial injury.

- <30% – <u>Recurrent back pain</u>. Individuals in this group have at least 2 or more reoccurrences of nearly identical pain in the exact same place. In the more problematic form of the disease, individuals can have 100's to even 1000's of reoccurrences (at different severity levels). Commonly, re-injury occurs at a certain activity level threshold (i.e., amount of weight lifted). However, in certain individuals re-injury can occur by simply taking a step wrong or during a mild twisting motion. Each reoccurrence (especially severe and moderate) can noticeably lower the activity level threshold at which the pain will reoccur. The most common form of therapy is decreasing the activity level to a progressively lower level (at least for a few months). This form of recurrent back strain affects at least 20-50 million people in the USA alone.

RECURRENT BACK STRAIN (MYOFASCIAL STRAIN)

Both how <u>long</u> it takes to heal a back strain and the <u>pain severity</u> are important in grouping the types and presentations of "recurrent back strain".

In over 2000 individuals questioned, most all had experienced some type of minimal injury. Minimal or mild injury or less was reported 50% of the time. Moderate injury occurred in another 30%. Severe strain in only 20% of those having back pain.

1. Minimal – Usually 1-2 hours maximum duration. Always less than one day duration.
   a. Stiff and sore. (Experienced by completely healthy muscles as well.) [Note: Can be painful. Overactive individuals in the "never any back pain" group will report this as an episode of "severe" back pain.]
   b. "Zinger" – sharp shooting pain that last seconds. Can occur in the back or a shooting pain radiating down the front or side of the thigh. These always occur above the level of the knee. Pain extending below the knee can often represent a serious sciatic nerve problem.

2. Mild – Lasting 1-2 days and rapidly resolves.

3. Moderate – Lasting 2-5 days and resolves over 1-2 weeks. After the first 2-3 reoccurrences many never seek medical attention. These individuals usually simply deal with the problem. The majority reported 1-5 years before the pain would reoccur. Commonly seen as a first presentation of back pain in teenagers.

4. Severe – Lasting 1-2 months before feeling near normal. Often the patient will report that they "<u>never did return to normal</u>" after that injury. The pain is often so severe the individual cannot walk normally for 1-2 weeks. A comfortable position cannot be found either standing or lying down. Simple activities like getting dressed or putting on shoes can often take 15 minutes due to pain and immobility. The pain intensity is described as one of the most severe pains that the individual has ever experienced. It is often compared with the pain experienced with a broken bone or major surgery. The initial episode is frequently followed by a series of mild and moderate episodes. Generally not seen before age 20.
   a. <u>Presentations of Severe Strain</u>:
      1. Severe immediate onset: Immediate onset of pain usually associated with a distinct activity (frequently heavy lifting or heavy lifting while twisting). This is the most common presentation of the first episode of back pain.
      2. Mild pain, then progressive: Immediate onset of only a mild pain, similar to a pulled muscle. Every 2 hours the pain progresses in severity. Over a 6-8 hour period, the pain progresses to the level of severe pain.

3. **Mild pain until twisting: Mild to moderate pain can exist for up to 1-2 days. However, with a slight twisting motion, the pain instantly goes to a severe level.**

Stretching exercises can be a very powerful tool. There is an old saying, "to a man with a hammer, everything looks like a nail". Certain mild acute injuries can appear similar to a chronically injured muscle. <u>Acute injuries</u> **do not respond** to intense stretching techniques. Trying to stretch acute injuries can prolong healing and even make the injury worse. It is analogous to attempting to stretch a badly sprained ankle. The muscles must be allowed to heal to a certain level before stretching techniques are of value.

A common scenario is that after a few weeks or months with the Opti-stretch technique people report "feeling better". This sensation of "feeling better" often results in an increase of activity level. There is even a tendency for these individuals to increase activity levels very significantly. If they progress too rapidly without first conditioning the muscles, mild injuries are common. After overdoing the day before, they may awaken the next morning feeling fine. However, on reaching for something or moving differently, they notice muscle discomfort. A common response is to think, "there's a muscle I haven't used in a day or two". Frequently it is a stiff and sore muscle that will improve with gentle stretching and slow progressive movement. It generally improves within 1 to 2 hours. However, this injury could be a mild acute injury that may be made worse with aggressive stretching techniques. Often these acute injuries are only discovered while doing the stretching exercises. Therefore, the injury is attributed to the stretching technique while in actuality the injury occurred the day before. For this reason, a gentle detection phase is performed to make certain there are no acutely injured muscles.

There are some general guidelines for determining mild and moderate acute muscle strains. The most common way to gauge an acute injury is by the amount of pain or discomfort. While this type of scale is useful to the individual, not everyone's scale is the same. For example, a strain causing severe pain to a six-year-old might be described as mild pain by a 16-year-old. To a 26-year-old professional football player, the exact same strain might be considered to be in the mild discomfort range.

A helpful approach is to compare the acute or chronically injured muscle with a normal healthy muscle. There are several general types of "stretch-to-pain" transitions for muscle tissue. Healthy muscles have intensity of discomfort characterized by 4 recognizable points between "no sensation of any stretch" and the sensation of pain (see Graph 1, page 88). This allows 4 recognizable levels of discomfort. With any type of muscle tissue that is not healthy, the transition ranges are significantly shorted to the point that they are not recognizable by the individual. Different groups of muscles have slightly different transitions. For instance, the muscles of the neck respond very differently to stretch than do the larger core muscles of the hips and low back. While muscle groups vary, the muscles of a single group on either side of the body should not. If indeed the "stretch-to-pain" transitions do vary, this suggests that a muscle with a more rapid transition toward pain is not as healthy compared to the other paired muscle. By utilizing stretching exercises to tone the muscles, the muscles can again return to a healthy state. When the muscles regain their healthy state, pathologic conditions (i.e., shortened tendon) can be determined. If a tendon has indeed shortened, there is no good treatment for this condition except to maintain exceptionally healthy muscles in that particular muscle group.

Muscles with tendon shortening appear to have more problems with healing properly than muscles without tendon shortening. The problem appears in part to be one of pure physics. A shortened tendon produces more stress on the muscle. This is seldom a significant clinical factor, if muscles are healthy. However, in a muscle that is unhealthy (poorly toned), this stress leads to increased fatigue of the muscle. This condition makes the muscle more susceptible to an injury than its paired muscle on the other side of the body.

Prior to the 1980's, there were no clinical diagnoses for the many chronic pain syndromes which physicians now recognize. Some physicians previously thought the condition to be "all in the person's head". The discovery of pathologic states causing disorders like chronic back pain, fibromyalgia, reflex sympathetic dystrophy and many others, led to the field of Chronic Pain Management, better known as "Pain Management", (which I happened to specialize in). The working definition of chronic pain is pain that persists beyond two months without improvement. As a field of medicine, Pain Management is very new.

"Recurrent back strain" is not considered a Chronic Pain Diagnosis. However in the most severe form, it becomes very similar to the diagnosis of Chronic Back Pain. Anyone who has severely pulled a low back muscle will often report that the injury bothered them for two to six months or even a year before they considered themselves back to normal. Even then, that identical back injury would again crop up several years later. This scenario is extremely common. These **irritated** muscles behave clinically similar to ACIMs, except that the individual can feel some type of discomfort or mild pain in the muscle. In the ACIMs the chronically injured muscle is present but "asymptomatic". Whether this condition can transform into a true "chronic pain syndrome" is unknown. It is generally believed not to occur. However, for individuals over age 40, the severe form of a "recurrent back pain syndrome", can cause near daily discomfort and significant limitations to physical activities. The condition can closely mimic certain chronic pain medical syndromes.

Illustrated below are 3 general muscle types and their respective stretch-to-pain transitions. Keep in mind that both irritated muscles in various stages of healing, and poorly toned muscles, behave very similar to the ACIMs.

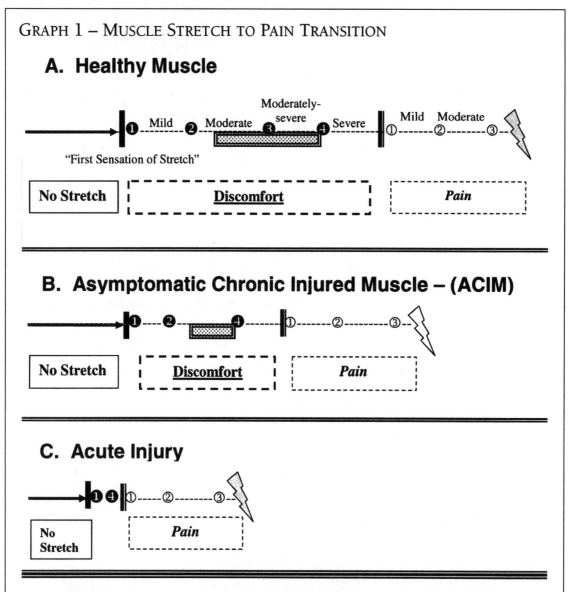

> ▶ ▦▦▦▦ - "Stretch receptor lengthening". A narrow and variable window.
> ▶ In a large **Healthy Muscle**, four different points of discomfort during stretched range-of-motion can be identified before the onset of pain.
> ▶ In both an **ACIM** or **Poorly Toned Muscle**, less than four points of discomfort can be felt and the distance of stretch between these points are shortened. Segment three - ❸, the "Moderately-severe Discomfort Range" is frequently absent. The other segments are shortened giving the clinical sensation of a tighter muscle.
> ▶ In an **Acute Injury**, the "first sensation of stretch" occurs sooner. Clinically, movement beyond the first sensation of stretch, results in that of "Pain". As the muscle injury heals, gradual increasing of the "**Discomfort**" range occurs.

Graph 2 – Male Stretch to Pain Transition

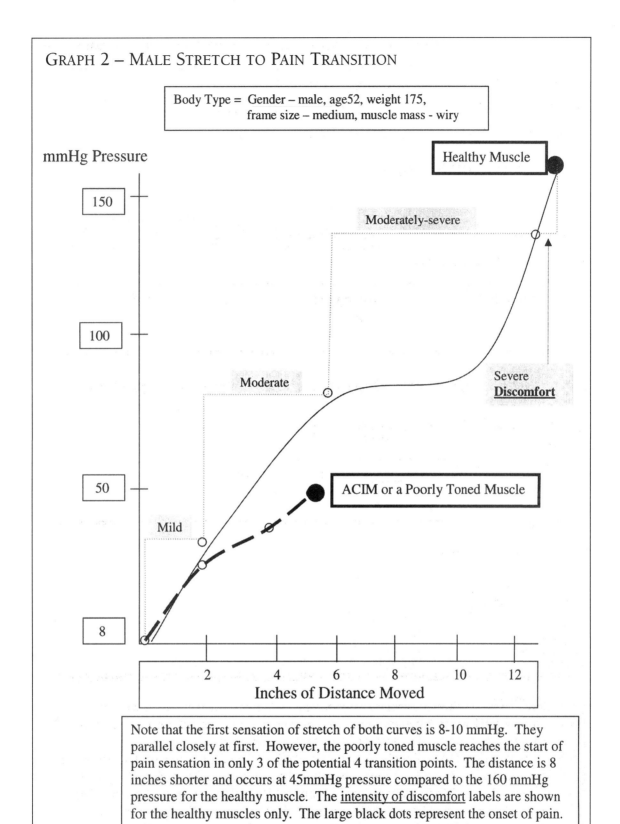

Body Type = Gender – male, age 52, weight 175, frame size – medium, muscle mass - wiry

mmHg Pressure

Healthy Muscle

150

Moderately-severe

100

Moderate

Severe **Discomfort**

50

ACIM or a Poorly Toned Muscle

Mild

8

2   4   6   8   10   12

Inches of Distance Moved

Note that the first sensation of stretch of both curves is 8-10 mmHg. They parallel closely at first. However, the poorly toned muscle reaches the start of pain sensation in only 3 of the potential 4 transition points. The distance is 8 inches shorter and occurs at 45mmHg pressure compared to the 160 mmHg pressure for the healthy muscle. The intensity of discomfort labels are shown for the healthy muscles only. The large black dots represent the onset of pain.

<u>Again</u>, don't stretch an <u>acutely injured muscle</u>. Give the muscle at least 2 to 5 days before gradually resuming gentle stretching exercises. Moderate strains may need 5 to 7 days or more. Only at a certain point in the healing phase will acutely injured muscles respond to stretching techniques. Daily stretching can actually prolong the healing phase due to daily irritation of the acute injury (like picking off a scab). Don't worry about lost progress.

Intensity of Stretch

"More is not better!" This is commonly referred to the "just right phenomenon" or the "Goldie Locks phenomenon". If you are stretching with the proper breathing technique and the proper incremental-movement technique, either too little or too much intensity will slow your progress. Any comfortable level where you are still seeing progressive stretch receptor lengthening and general well being of the muscle, is an adequate intensity level. However, some will try to press the envelope (press to more extreme intensity levels). If you think of your daily stretches as significantly uncomfortable, you are probably stretching with too extreme of an intensity level. If you are feeling any <u>residual stretch</u> or discomfort in the muscles after stopping the stretching exercise, this is a dangerous level. It is defined as stretching in the severe discomfort range. While it is not recommended, some individuals try to learn where this level is. If they stay just under this level, this is considered the moderately-severe range. This is considered to be the maximum safe level of stretching intensity. Most stretching exercises only require a moderate discomfort level.

Only Intermediate exercises "Sitting Nose to Knee" – (Figure Four) and "Supine Straight Knee to Nose" should be used in this moderately-severe range. For learning purposes, the "Sitting Knees to Floor" – (Butterfly) can be used to experience sensitive muscles, which can be most safely pushed into the <u>residual stretch</u> range. It is imperative not to enter this range with any of the more central core muscles of the back.

Your intensity level is too extreme if any of the following occur.

1. Any sensation of residual stretch.
2. Any stiffness or soreness the following day.
3. Repeating a stretch and the level of moderate discomfort is reached noticeably sooner than the time before.

Step #3 of the Opti-stretch Challenge (Maintenance Program)

■ ■ ■

> If you are a fit athlete or child, try the Advanced Program.

Congratulations, this is the final step of the Opti-stretch Challenge. The Therapeutic Program used stretch receptor lengthening for new range. The Maintenance Program simply preserves this new found optimum range of motion, even into advanced age.

Some may have slightly overshot their optimum range of motion in order to properly tone ACIMs. Therefore, the Maintenance Program range of motion could be somewhat slightly less, as-long-as movement on both sides are symmetrical. This way, the Maintenance Program becomes time-efficient and designed for decades of continual use.

Some enjoy performing these exercises on a daily basis. Many find it relaxing and invigorating at the start or end of their day. Others, like myself, prefer not having to perform daily stretches. By understanding the physiology presented in this book, good warm up techniques prior to high activity levels can also be used to preserve muscle tone and avoid injury. If the later is chosen, a weekly level of complex movement activity needs to designed. Different activities for the different seasons of the year work well.

For example, after completing the Intermediate Program, the activity I chose was swimming. It requires complex range of motion while at the same time strengthens and conditions the body. During rests, the "Kneeling Back Bridge", "Squat", and "Finger Touch" can be easily performed in the water to make sure that all the major muscle groups are exercised. The more complex motion the activity has, the less need for daily stretching.

I started the Maintenance Program, when I was able to obtain equal range of motion on both sides. If unable to achieve this range of motion in 3 sets, I usually restart daily stretching for a week or two. Then, I try every other day stretching. After a couple weeks, every third day is tried. For the first year, twice a week or weekly tests should be performed to make sure you can still comfortably reach your optimum range of motion.

No matter what type of maintenance program you choose, the most important goal is to maintain your optimum range of motion. The best way to achieve this, is to have fun. Muscle physiology is very dynamic. This makes it enjoyable to perform periodic tests, to evaluate how the muscles are doing. Also, if this level of range of motion is not maintained, my back seems a little stiff; activities start becoming more uncomfortable and fatiguing. One of the last things I want, is returning to the vicious cycle of a "bad back".

Opti-stretch Advanced Program for Fit Athletes and Children

■ ■ ■

1. Sitting Nose to Knee – (Figure Four)
2. Sitting Knees to Floor – (Butterfly)
3. Standing Squat
4. Bridge
5. Kneeling Back Bridge
6. Supine Ankles to Pelvis
7. Supine Feet Apart
8. Prone Knee to Cross Chest
9. Second Position
10. Butterfly Extreme Scissors

> Note:
> The Advanced Program is to be used only as a screening test. Not all of the exercises are designed for daily use.

While the Advanced Program is quite simple for children and fit athletes, it can be very physically demanding for older individuals. For this reason a physical exam is needed beyond age 35 and those with any medical illness should not perform these exercises. For those who can, the exercises represent an excellent benchmark for muscle tone. Most are checked periodically. The Intermediate Program is designed to prepare you.

I perform the "Bridge" a couple times a month. It should be noted that in some university swimming programs, the "Bridge" is now discouraged for daily use, because "it can hurt the back". There are many exercises like this that have been discouraged or even stopped in public physical education classes for this reason. However, certain individuals can perform these exercises daily without ever hurting their backs. This suggests that it is not the exercise, but the baseline muscle tone of the individual. If psoas muscles are targeted using extreme exercises, before first toning the surrounding larger muscles, this can definitely lead to back pain (i.e., the bent-knee sit-up with the hands behind the head, and using a jerking motion can put a tremendous stress directly on the psoas muscles).

The "Standing Squat" is the one single exercise that seems to have the highest correlation with having a healthy back (especially in men). I perform it daily, but still have trouble with it due to tightened soleus muscles (in the calf), and the shortened psoas tendon.

The "Prone Knee to Cross Chest" is excellent and can be used instead of other pyriformis stretches. Tested regularly are the "Supine Feet Apart", and the "Second Position". However, the "Supine Ankles to Pelvis" is diagnostic only and can cause knee pain with daily use.

1. SITTING NOSE TO KNEE – (FIGURE FOUR)

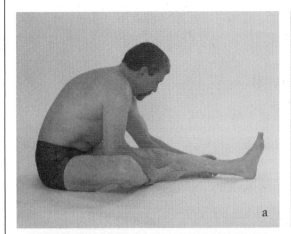
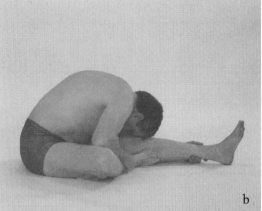

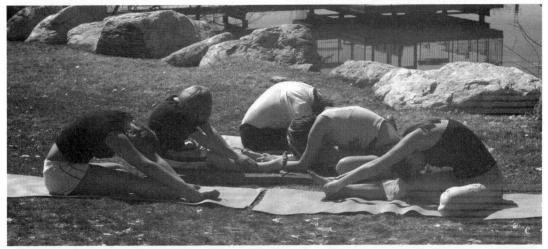

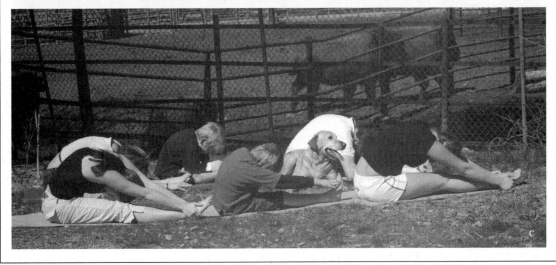

1. SITTING NOSE TO KNEE – (FIGURE FOUR) (CONTINUED)

a. Sit with the left leg extended. The right knee is bent with the arch of the right foot touching the bulge on the inside of the left knee.
b. Slowly touch the nose to the knee.
c. Individuals, ages 8 to 51, are shown in this figure.

Notes:
1. Repeat for the right side of the body.
2. This should be both a relatively easy position to obtain and quite comfortable. Both the left and right stretches should be to equal length.
3. You should be able to at least bring the nose within 4 inches of the knee before proceeding on to the rest of the advanced stretches.
4. Often in Yoga, the left foot is placed against the right thigh. In martial arts, the left foot is placed on the calf. If you are used to one way, still perform the stretch as described in Opti-stretch with the arch of the left foot over the bulge of the right knee. This has been found to be the best way to tone the hamstrings for further Opti-stretch exercises.

2. SITTING KNEES TO FLOOR – (BUTTERFLY)

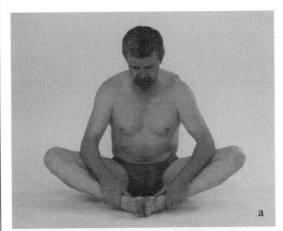
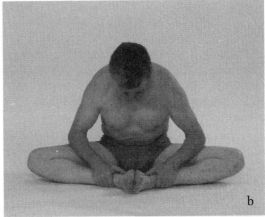

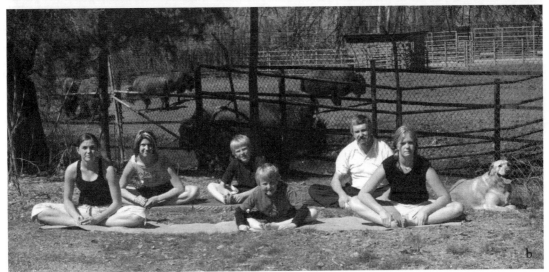

a. In the sitting position bring the soles of the feet together. Grasp the ankles. Rest the elbows on the thighs close to the knees.

b. Exert pressure on the thighs by using the elbows. Slowly place the legs flat on the floor.

Notes:
1. Knees should be at least 4 inches from the floor before proceeding on to the other Advanced stretches.

3. Standing Squat – psoas major and minor muscles

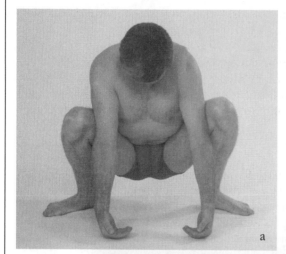
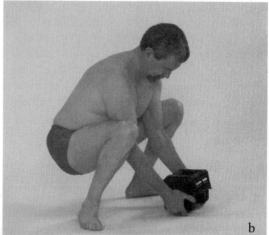

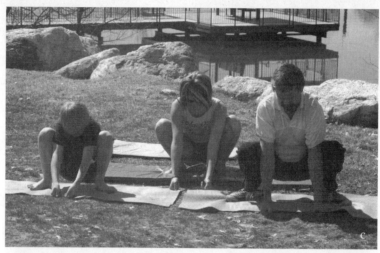

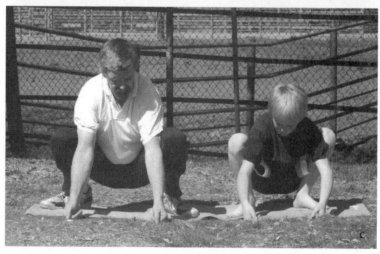

3. STANDING SQUAT – PSOAS MAJOR AND MINOR MUSCLES (CONTINUED)

a. Stand in a slightly wide leg stance and squat down. Pretend you are lifting a small heavy box off the floor using an optimum lifting technique.

b. If there is ankle tightness sometimes the feet need to be rotated to the outside. Still you should be in a stable position to lift something if you needed to.

c. This is an extremely simple stretching exercise for children. In many foreign countries the majority of 60-80 year old individuals can get comfortably into this resting position and sit for hours. If you cannot comfortably touch the hands to the floor, you by definition have to be <u>lifting with your back</u> instead of your legs.

Notes:

1. This is the <u>most dangerous</u> of the Opti-stretch Stretching Exercises.

2. While simple for many, those who are unable to comfortably achieve this position can experience the following: functional compression of the aorta or vena cava causing transient high blood pressure or dizziness on standing up. It is believed to be responsible for dislodging blood clots in individuals prone to blood clots.

3. Always have an <u>experienced spotter</u> to help you before attempting this position.

4. Unfortunately, this is an extremely important stretching exercise. If you are healthy enough to work on it and finally achieve full range of motion you will be able to note a difference in how healthy your back muscles are.

4. Bridge – Psoas Muscle Complex

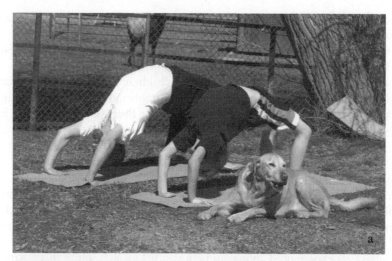

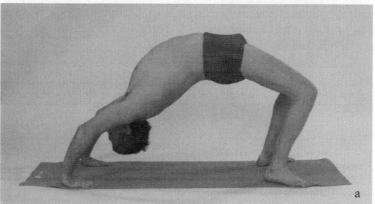

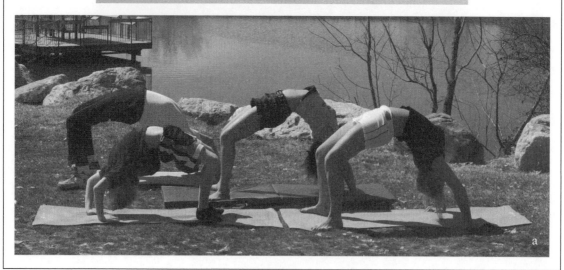

4. BRIDGE – PSOAS MUSCLE COMPLEX (CONTINUED)

a. While lying on the back place your hands over your head and place the hands close to the shoulders and flat on the floor. Using the strength of the arms, slowly arch the back into the air. Often it is necessary to reposition the arms while resting some weight on the head. When repositioned, using only the arms, elevate the body into the bridge position.

Notes:
1. Always use a <u>qualified spotter</u>! The spotter should not help by lifting the body. They should only protect you from falling if your hands slip.
2. By age 3, most all children can easily perform this stretching exercise. Many sports such as swimming, diving, gymnastics and dance regularly teach 3 year olds this exercise.
3. Only about 50% of school age children can perform this exercise. Only 20% of adults can perform this.
4. This exercise significantly stretches the psoas muscle complex of the low back. The exercise is particularly hard to do with recurrent back problems.
5. Additionally, good range of motion of the wrists and shoulders is essential. Some individuals will have adequate range of motion of the low back but due to wrist and shoulder problems will have difficulty with this exercise.
6. Upper body strength to body weight ratio is also accessed.
7. It is a great exercise if your joints are healthy.
8. This is not intended as a daily exercise but as a check to evaluate the above muscles and joints usually 2 –3 times per month.

5. KNEELING BACK BRIDGE – PSOAS COMPLEX MUSCLES

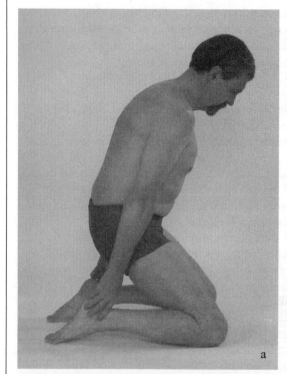

a

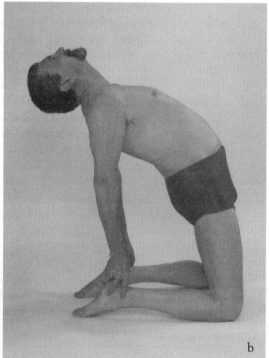

b

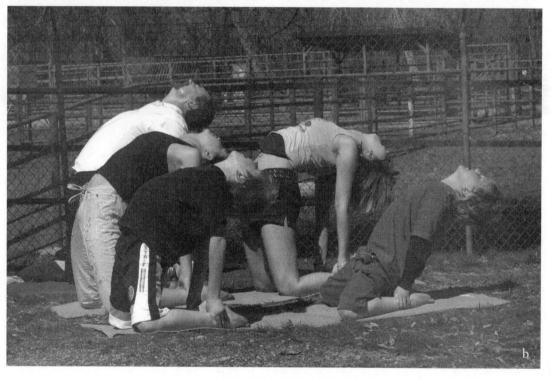

b

5. KNEELING BACK BRIDGE – PSOAS COMPLEX MUSCLES (CONTINUED)

a.   In the kneeling position, place your hands on the back side of the ankles.
b.   Arch the back forward and upward. This places a significant stretch on the psoas muscles.

Notes:
1.   This does not put quite as much stretch on the psoas muscles as does the normal bridge position.
2.   For individuals with shoulder and wrist problems this is a preferable stretching exercise.
3.   Perform slowly and carefully. Still use an experienced spotter, as it is quite easy to lose your balance with this stretching exercise. This especially is true in the early learning phase.

6. Supine Ankles to Pelvis – (Diagnostic Stretch Only)

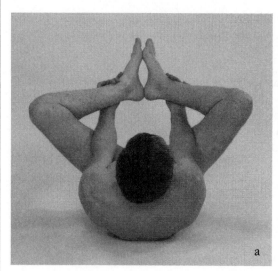 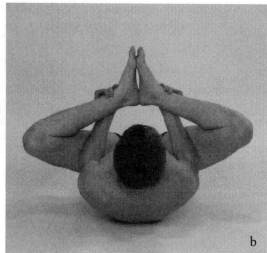

a.   In the supine position, grasp the legs near the ankles. Use an underhand grip.

b.   Slowly and gently bring the heels toward the pelvis or groin area.

Notes:

1.   Be cautious not to strain the knees with this stretching exercise.

2.   This particular stretching exercise can put tremendous strain on the low back. Be very careful.

3.   If there is a rapid transition from mild stretch to significant discomfort in the low back, there is a good possibility you may have tight iliopsoas and psoas complex muscles.

4.   If this stretching exercise reproduces your low back discomfort you need to seriously consider the full 6 months of Opti-stretch Intermediate Therapeutic Program and obtaining the maximum levels of range of motion. **This stretch is used for diagnosis and not for daily use due to the excess stress on the knees.**

7. SUPINE FEET APART – ADDUCTOR MUSCLES

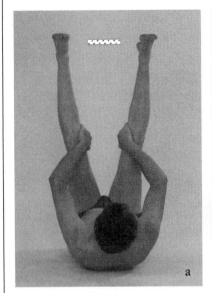 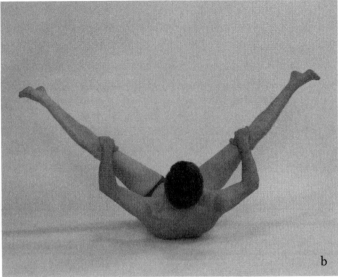

a. In the supine position use the arms to spread the feet apart. The distance apart of the feet can be measured.

b. Extra stretch can be applied by using the arms to pull the shoulders and upper body slightly forward.

Note:

1. While this is the safest way and best way to perform the stretch in the beginning, once the adductors have been sufficiently toned, other more effective ways of stretching the adductors can be experimented with.

2. My personal preference is the standing stretch. The legs are horizontal and wide apart. The right adductor is stretched by keeping the right leg and hip straight while the left knee is slowly bent. The hands are on the floor for support.

8. PRONE KNEE TO CROSS CHEST – PYRIFORMIS STRETCH

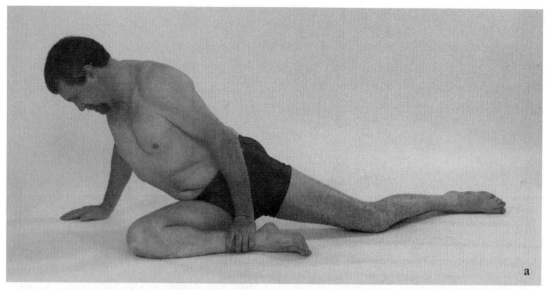

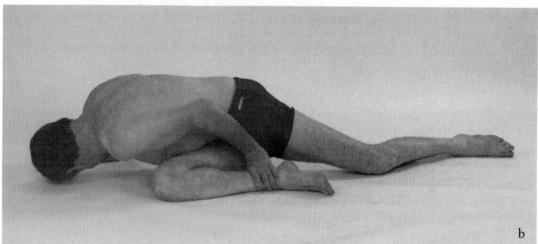

a. In the cheerleader position with the back leg fully extended, grab either the right ankle or knee with the left hand.

b. Controlling the weight of the upper body with the arms, slowly allow the right knee and left shoulder to touch. (Knee to the cross shoulder).

Notes:
1. This is designed to stretch all the 6 hip flexor muscles of which the pyriformis is the one most commonly recognized.
2. By putting the left hand beneath the right knee and gently pulling, you may place extra stretch on the hip flexor muscles.
3. Occasionally, return to the "Supine Knee to Cross Chest" and "Sitting Knee to Cross Chest" to assure all the hip flexors are being sufficiently stretched.

9. SECOND POSITION

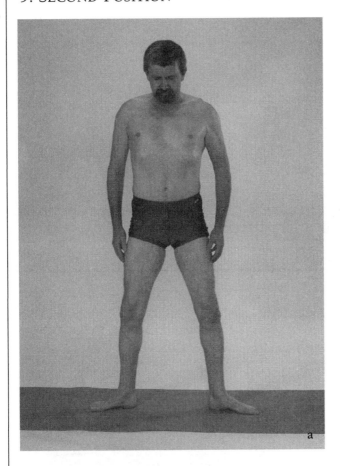

a. This is a common dance position. With the knees bent and the feet approximately shoulder width, rotate the feet so the toes are pointing 180 degrees from each other. Slowly tighten the quadriceps until the knees are straight.

Note:
1. This requires a great deal of strength of the gluteus medius muscle. Discomfort of one side of the back and upper pelvic area is a risk factor. Also rotation of the pelvis is considered to be a risk factor. Use the various muscles of the pelvis to try and prevent rotation.

10. Butterfly Extreme Scissors – Sartorias and Gracilis

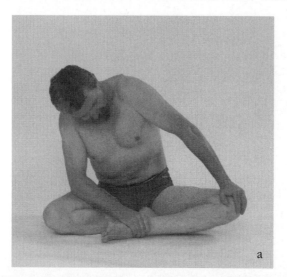

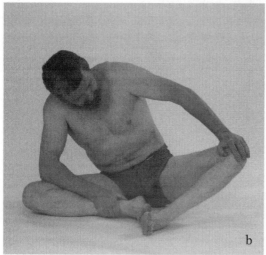

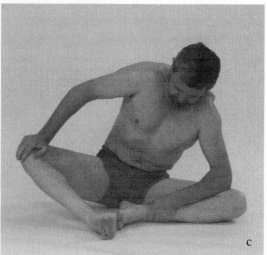

a. The extreme scissors differs from the (Butterfly) in that the right foot is drawn as close to the groin as possible. The left foot crosses midline. In this position, the stretch focuses on two muscles that are commonly tightened following certain knee injuries. If you have sustained a knee injury or have had trouble healing a knee strain, this can be a very valuable stretching exercise. It is imperative to be extremely careful and gentle while even getting into the starting position.

b. In the beginning phases of this stretch, the left foot may need to be placed closer to midline until the thigh muscles become more toned.

c. This shows the position for stretching the right knee.

SUMMARY OF THE OPTI-STRETCH PROGRAM

■ ■ ■

A major accomplishment of the Opti-stretch Program was to demonstrate that certain individuals, over time, can regain a certain range of motion. This improved range of motion and subsequent conditioning of back muscles leads to a significant decrease in muscular back strain, and increase in both activity levels and athletic ability. The application of this knowledge can be of extreme benefit to the benign back pain sufferer (especially those suffering from moderate and severe pain syndromes).

Some people believe that the Opti-stretch goals of optimum range of motion to the level of the "gold standard" with certain stretching exercises are possibly too extreme. These specific goals are provided as stopping point goals. If a person suffers from poor posture or a recurrent back problem, he or she may have to obtain such levels before they can honestly say that no stone has been left unturned. Stretching beyond these levels has not demonstrated any significant improvement in back health.

Even with exercising the limited asymmetric side twice as much as the more flexible side, many do not reach symmetry and complete toning of the muscles until close to these optimal ranges-of-motion. Assuming that you had to work and develop at least 2 or more inches of stretch receptor lengthening to reach this optimal level, there is probably little to be gained by pushing the range of motion further. Hence, these ranges are optimal for most people. This provides both a stopping place to reside at <u>and</u> a realistic level to maintain for life.

Remember two things. First, there are individuals in their 60's and 70's that can do these stretches without any difficulty at all. Next, there is greater than a 90% chance that as a healthy child, you were doing all of these stretches on a regular basis while playing. This means your body at one time had been conditioned to do these stretches. It is far easier to regain a previous level of stretch than to push to new extremes. If you couldn't do these stretches as a child, you will be unlikely to reach this level as an adult. This knowledge gives you some realistic goals to strive for. Obviously with certain severe injuries and medical conditions, these goals may not be realistic. Other more reasonable goals then must be substituted.

Opti-stretch combines incremental breathing techniques, incremental movement techniques and certain therapeutic intensity force levels in order to provide optimal toning of the essential core muscles required to lift heavy objects. You are more than welcome to add additional stretching exercises to your own daily routine after completing the two to six month program. Remember, do not use the Opti-stretch Therapeutic Technique on any stretching exercise that is not included in this book. Another exciting part of the program is that it provides an excellent basis for evaluating the health of the back and the back muscles for an entire lifetime.

Individuals, who are hyperflexible and find these stretches too simple, need to pay particular attention to body symmetry differences. In addition, more specific stretches may need to be devised for this group of individuals to adequately assess basic health of the back. This is discussed later in the Scientific Consideration section #9: Hyperflexibility and Double-jointedness.

Once the basic Opti-stretch routine has achieved <u>either</u> symmetry <u>or</u> optimum range of motion, it is necessary to strengthen these muscles by at least 10-15%. There are many good published programs and sports trainers that can provide this knowledge. The final step of regaining optimum muscle health is to choose a good conditioning program. The easiest way involves some type of enjoyable sport.

There are certain sports that require performing an even more excessive range of motion than the optimum levels recommended by Opti-stretch. While this type of excessive range of motion has been implicated in causing certain problems, it has never been scientifically proven to be detrimental. However, while these excessive ranges-of-motion are advantageous in a given sport, they have never proven to be markedly beneficial in maintaining healthy muscles or joints. If you want to pursue excessive range of motion, first strive to obtain a good healthy set of core muscles at the Opti-stretch "gold standard" level. Some individuals make the mistake of pressing on to extremes of a given range of motion before first assuring a healthy set of core muscles. This can lead to developing significant body asymmetry.

Body asymmetry is extremely common in young girls. The parents will say, "look how flexible she is; she can even do the splits". On closer assessment, the girl will be able to comfortably do the splits with say the right leg forward. However, she may be able to go only half way down in completing the splits with the opposite leg forward. This is a classic example of body asymmetry and a risk factor for injuring the core muscles of the back. Remember that people with extreme range of motion often have as many <u>or even more</u> back problems than someone with very poor or limited range of motion. <u>Absolute range-of-motion</u> is not the key. **<u>The key is an optimal range of motion for your given body type.</u>** Opti-stretch is designed to help you both recognize this goal and achieve it. Eventually, the forces of nature such as aging, injury or disease will limit this ability. Hopefully, this will be long past the age of 85. Even then, you will still be at your optimum and that is generally the best you can realistically hope for.

WALKING PROGRAM

■ ■ ■

Don't forget to include a walking program for cardiovascular fitness. A 20 minute a day program can be performed in 5 minute intervals. The first 2 minutes should be a gentle warm-up walk. In 1 to 5 minute intervals, a brisk walk should be alternated with a lengthened stride walk. Pay careful attention with the lengthened stride walk to observe for any tightness in the groin area of one leg. Be careful not to overextend the stride too much and strain the groin area (iliopsoas). By gradually lengthening the stride, a significant portion of the psoas muscle on the affected side is both strengthened and conditioned.

PROGRESS CAREFULLY TO NEW ACTIVITY LEVELS

The major goal of Opti-stretch is to return to your optimum activity level. It is imperative to have your cardiovascular system equally as healthy as your back. There is a very serious potential problem, which I've seen both in students and myself. Despite months or years of inactivity due to back pain, once the back feels great, there is a tendency to immediately return to a previous activity level and even try to press further. While your new back may tolerate this, other skeletal structures and your heart may not. For example, at age 45, I had not lifted anything heavier than 60 pounds for 7 years. After completing the Opti-stretch program, I went to the gym to test my new back out. It felt very exhilarating to be lift heavy objects again. Before long, I was up to 250 pounds before straining a left hamstring muscle. I didn't even think about how much stress I was placing on my heart. This could have resulted in a more serious problem than just pulling a hamstring. Fortunately, I had been doing the walking program.

Remember, it is important to work up to your new activity levels gradually and intelligently. This is particularly true if you are over age 35, or if it has been more than a month since you had to stop a certain activity level.

Don't forget your heart and cardiovascular system while working at the Opti-stretch program. If you get the same near miraculous results that others have, a good healthy heart will come in handy to keep up with your new back.

Section II –
Scientific Considerations

■ ■ ■

1. Basics of Back Strain
2. Contraction vs. Spasm
3. Bone Spicules and Muscle Healing
4. Chronically Injured Muscles
5. Muscle Tone
6. Stretch Receptors
7. Involuntary Stretching – (Instinctive Stretching)
8. Range of Motion
9. Hyperflexibility and Double-Jointedness
10. Proprioceptive Neuromuscular Facilitation (PLF)
11. Acute Muscle Injury
12. Warming-up
13. The Psoas Short Leg Syndrome
14. The Psoas Muscle
    a. Anatomy
    b. Physiology
    c. Pain from the Psoas Muscle
    d. Function with Spasm
    e. Case Studies Evaluated with Opti-stretch Screening Exercises
15. Upper Back Pain and the Rhomboid Muscles
16. Neck Pain and the Trapezius Muscles
17. Shoulder Height and Asymmetry
18. Chiropractic and other Manipulations
19. Dyspareunia
20. Arthritis
21. Posture
22. "Dr. Mom"
23. Conclusion

1. BASICS OF BACK STRAIN

The two muscles of major interest are the psoas muscle of the low back and the rhomboid muscles of the upper back. These two core muscle groups are responsible for the majority of recurrent back strain episodes. Different methods to best rehabilitate these muscles were experimented with. Stretching exercises proved beneficial, not only for improving tone, but also for isolating the muscle or muscle groups. This allowed a system for determining risk factors. It also allowed for being able to measure accurately the increase in muscle tone.

The Advanced Program was developed. It is a collection of special complex exercises that certain active individuals, under the age of 35, could do rather easily. This group was also unique in that the majority had never experienced any type of significant back pain in their entire lives. In contrast, individuals who suffered from a history of recurrent back problems were unable to complete these stretching exercises. The exam was evaluated on individuals between the ages of 3 and 73. Over 95% of all healthy "3 to 5" year olds could pass these screening exercises. The percentage then falls precipitously over each half decade of life.

The Advanced Program was designed around the knowledge of the "never any back pain" group. Regarding the general population, these stretching exercises seem extremely simple to some; to others, they appear rather impossible. Indeed, from an anatomy and physiology point of view, these stretching exercises are rather complex. There are multiple reasons why an individual may not be able to pass the exam; some have nothing to do with the back. However, those who could pass the exam, demonstrated a much lower incidence of back problems in all age groups, especially age 35 and above. Those who could not pass the Advanced Program the first time around, due to back problems, and then worked on the Intermediate Therapeutic Program for 2 to 6 months were pleased. By the time they could pass the Advanced Program, many had noted significant decreases in their back pain problems. A long term, less demanding maintenance program could then be implemented.

The Opti-stretch therapeutic programs for old and young use the best stretching exercises out of more than 350 published stretching exercises. The technique of stretch receptor lengthening should only be used on the stretching exercises presented in this book. The technique must be performed very precisely, in order to both achieve optimum results and to avoid possible injury to the muscles. As muscles become more toned, it has been demonstrated that joint movement and posture can improve. The new measurement techniques are simple, yet extremely accurate. This allows for better tracking of progress, which assures that the individual is performing the therapeutic programs properly. It also aids in goal setting, and makes the stretching exercises more informative and fun.

Stretching exercises in Western Cultures have only become popular in the last 65 years. Some Middle Eastern and Eastern cultures have experience with stretching techniques that date back over 2000 years. Stretching exercises have proven to be a valuable tool to help maintain muscle tone and for helping to warm up muscles (especially in individuals over age 35).

In the USA, most individuals who are presently under the age of 55 have received at least some instruction, in either school classes or sports as to the value of stretching. Unfortunately, many learn to stretch with excessive intensity of force that actually inhibits stretch receptor lengthening, promotes injury and causes a discomfort that makes stretching unappealing for later life. The precise incidence of individuals using some type of stretching program is difficult to determine. In the individuals questioned, the incidence was very low.

Two popular types of stretching programs in adults were found. First, was a daily program. This was popular in people who had sustained a musculo-skeletal back injury. However, they often reported muscle tightening and return of the back pain, if only a few days or weeks of regular exercise were missed. Second, was a stretching program performed prior to intense physical activity. These individuals are commonly referred to as "weekend warriors". Often their job responsibilities preclude an active lifestyle during the week. However, on the weekends and vacations, very physical activities like skiing, rock climbing or aggressive yard work are performed. A fairly high percentage of these "weekend warriors", over 35, have at least some type of either stretching or other warm-up program, prior to engaging in physical activity.

Hopefully, this widespread disinterest in stretching exercises by the general public will change when individuals discover the amount of important knowledge that can be gained by completing the Opti-stretch program. The therapeutic programs are designed for 20 minutes each day for 2 to 6 months. Unfortunately, the older the individual and the longer the muscles have had problems, the longer it takes to remedy the problem. The major goal is to correct risk factors for recurrent back strain. Once goals are reached, many find they can change to a 2 to 3 times per week program or even just periodic checks as a screening and diagnostic tool. A lot depends on the type of risk factors and the type of active lifestyle the individual maintains. If risk factors can be completely eliminated, muscle tone can often be maintained for prolonged periods by an active lifestyle and regaining "involuntary stretching" (see Section 7). It is important to at least periodically check to ensure the level of muscle tone is not decreasing.

The major goal of Opti-stretch is to detect unhealthy muscles and restore the proper elasticity and tone to the muscle fibers. An unhealthy muscle is one that has some element of tightness or spasm in the muscle. This is usually a residual effect of an injury to the muscle that has caused some degree of spasm in the muscle. Toning the muscles is only part of the process for maintaining healthy muscles. Once muscles are toned, the next two steps are to strengthen and condition the muscles. To review the next steps of strengthening and conditioning muscles, I completed a Certified Personal Fitness Trainer course. There are many excellent programs to choose from, in order to strengthen the muscles. Fewer programs deal with the conditioning of muscles, especially for amateurs and adults.

Good programs generally stress the importance of stretching. However, there doesn't appear to be any packaged program quite like Opti-stretch for both detecting risk factors and then effectively decreasing the risk factors through muscle toning.

Opti-stretch is a very new program. Because certain new medical discoveries contradicted generally accepted medical dogma, five years were spent working with these concepts and only on select individuals. All have noted improvement in back pain, muscle function and fewer recurrences of muscle strain. Some have experienced dramatic improvement and have even described the results as a "fountain of youth". The program was designed for both safety and efficiency. Because of the complexity of the stretching exercises, isolation of specific problematic muscles, and the new techniques used, injuries while performing the stretching exercises are still possible, if the basic concepts are not properly understood. The program must be followed very precisely to avoid injuries.

Opti-stretch was designed for essentially healthy individuals and those without significant medical problems. Anyone with medical problems, over the age of 35 or any history of serious back injuries needs to have a medical evaluation prior to even trying the program. For the past six years, I have experimented with aspects of this program. Many of the theories were tested and retested to assure long-term viability, time efficiency and safety. However, like many things in life, there are no guarantees. You need to be aware that there may be medical risks to certain types of individuals. Always read the exercise carefully before attempting any stretching exercise. An experienced fitness instructor is extremely beneficial. Unless you are generally healthy and accept that there may be risks in performing these stretching exercises, please do not attempt the exercises without an instructor.

Preventable recurrent back problems and risk factors <u>can be identified</u>. By maximizing muscle tone, many young and old alike can be spared the needless decrease in activity levels that can accompany "Benign Back Pain". Significant pain and suffering for millions of individuals can now be avoided. Please evaluate the Opti-stretch program. Any constructive criticism and ideas for future evolution of this new program are welcome.

2. CONTRACTION VS. SPASM

In science, the more that is understood about a problem, the better are the chances of a solution. Many times demonstrating theories to be wrong can be very beneficial when trying to solve very complex scientific problems. In the following sections, mainstream theories are simply presented as generally accepted scientific fact. Opti-stretch theories are clearly indicated so you will know these are still only theories. Other published theories are included, which for one reason or another have not been perpetuated in mainstream scientific literature.

Muscles are part of the musculo-skeletal organ system. Their physiology and function are very complex. As an organ, it is one of the few organs of the body that have two completely opposite functions. The first function is to contract and provide movement of the body. The second function is to spasm and specifically prevents movement of the body. This spasm or injury response is the same whether there is direct injury to the muscle or indirectly caused by pain stimuli from surrounding structures like joints, ligaments and bone.

During mild injury, an agonistic muscle will usually undergo partial spasm. When moderate injury occurs, not only the agonistic muscle but also the accessory muscles that serve the same function as the agonistic muscle will spasm. During a severe injury, like a broken femur (thighbone) of an animal, the antagonist muscles will also spasm. Simultaneous spasm of the primary muscles of movement, their accessory muscles, and the antagonistic muscles provide complete immobilization of the bone or joint. This complete immobilization allows for healing. If allowed to move, a broken bone will often not heal or will calcify in two separate pieces rather than one. This obviously is a serious complication. After sufficient healing of the bone, the majority of the time the muscles will gradually return to their normal function for movement of the limbs, especially where a muscle crosses only one joint. However, in certain core muscles, which can travel over 7 to 8 joints, there is an increased risk of chronic injury to those muscles.

3. Bone Spicules and Muscle Healing

A significant strain to a muscle causes injury to the individual muscle fibers. When there is clinical evidence of the injury like swelling or bruising, a strain is then referred to clinically, as a sprain. Because of the depth of the core muscles of the back, seldom does this type of clinical evidence manifest itself. Therefore, back strain, rather than back sprain, is usually diagnosed in most lifting injuries involving the back.

On a cellular level, when muscle tissue is damaged and pulled away from the bone, a healing process occurs much like healing a broken bone. Small needle-like fragments of bone tissue (spicules) are formed between the muscle fibers in the first few weeks following injury. Weeks later, the bone fragments are dissolved as scar tissue heals the injury. With strengthening of the muscle fibers, the muscle returns to essentially normal with the exception of various amounts of scar tissue formation. Unless the strain is extremely severe, seldom do peripheral muscles of the limbs have a tendency to become restrained. Usually, the healing process is 110%, which means there is very little chance of recurrent strain in that area of the muscle. In sharp contrast, certain core muscles commonly form asymptomatic chronically injured muscles (ACIMs), which have a very high rate of recurrent strain.

With a true <u>sprain</u> (anatomic damage), the individual experiences immediate severe pain in the muscle so that any movement causes further pain. In 5 to 7 days, the muscle will start to feel better and begins to allow movement. The range of motion of the muscle is usually still very limited. As the injury heals, movement gradually returns. There is also a change from immediate pain when the muscle is moved. As the muscle heals, some type of warning level of discomfort will occur. This warns that if there is any further stretch, pain will occur. Anyone who has sustained a severe muscle strain knows the last 1/2 inch of range of motion is always the hardest to heal and often takes months to completely heal. In this last 1/2 inch of range of motion, the muscle frequently undergoes several minor <u>reinjuries</u> or strains before total healing occurs. Frequently a month or two later, the exact same muscle injury can "act up" again. Some injuries can take six months to over a year before the muscles seem back to normal again.

Commonly, the muscle heals to where it functionally feels pretty good but the last 1/2 inch of range of motion has not yet returned. In limb muscles, this is usually quite obvious to the individual and in today's modern medicine, this limitation is generally unacceptable. Physical Therapy is usually prescribed and over time, the range of motion of the muscle and joint is usually returned to normal. In the core muscles (muscles of the spine, hips, neck, and shoulders) this last 1/2-inch of decreased range of motion frequently goes undetected. Unfortunately, the individual usually does not know the precise range of motion of these core muscles, prior to the injury. Therapists have broad ranges, which are considered normal. Therefore, when the pain stops and the muscle fells better, many still have not reached their own personal and preexisting range of motion.

Clinically, using most of today's standard methods, this difference in range of motion of core muscles can be very difficult to detect and evaluate. Also, the optimum range of motion varies quite significantly for each individual body type. Much of this individual variation appears to be genetically controlled. Also, there can be large variations due to environmental control. Therefore, certain core muscles can feel essentially normal but simply have not completely healed to the level of a healthy muscle and go completely unnoticed. This problem can last for decades, as you will see below.

4. CHRONICALLY INJURED MUSCLES

Core muscles of the body can remain in a state of partial spasm for long periods of time, such as years. This muscle state is referred to as a chronically injured muscle, when the individual has some indication of discomfort at rest or during an activity. In medicine, this is often seen in individuals who continually push a significantly injured muscle and not allow it to heal properly. Many individuals with significant injuries, due to something like a car accident, have reported over a year to heal the muscle and another 3 to 4 years to get the muscle feeling back to essentially normal.

The asymptomatic chronically injured muscle (ACIM) behaves exactly the same, except that the individual is completely unaware that there is a problem. Four T's characterize this condition:

1. Tightness to stretch,
2. Tenderness to touch,
3. Trigger points (a name for knots in the muscle that are especially tender),
4. Transition of stretch to pain is shortened.

To the individual, the muscle is asymptomatic and usually seems to function about the same as it used to, prior to the injury. However, the muscle is extremely susceptible to reinjury and recurrent strains. These asymptomatic chronically injured muscles (ACIMs) are more noticeable in the upper back and neck muscles because the core muscles involved are quite superficial. Frequently, these muscles do not completely heal when treated by normal physical therapy treatment. In the 1960's, Dr. Janet Travell, personal physician to Presidents Kennedy and Johnson, first demonstrated that trigger points could be injected with various medications. This promoted healing in many individuals. However, in some individuals, the symptoms would simply resolve for two weeks and then return. Healing any type of chronically injured muscle still remains a difficult task in medicine.

Opti-stretch has demonstrated that asymptomatic chronically injured muscles (ACIMs), even without knots, exhibit some degree of tenderness. Often the muscle tenderness is so slight that it can only be detected by putting precisely the same amount of pressure simultaneously on the chronically injured muscle and the healthy muscle located on the other side of the body. The same exact force to each side of the body usually allows the individual to detect the slight increase in tenderness or tightness. Frequently, massage therapists will point out these tight and tender muscles to the individual. Many massage therapists will then encourage stretching exercises for the individual. Other types of "therapists" may recommend a myofascial release or more invasive type of therapy.

The Opti-stretch screening stretches are designed specifically for the average individual to be able to confirm what their massage therapist has told them. They can detect these tight and tender muscles for themselves. Patho-physiologically, these muscles appear not to have undergone complete healing (cross webbing of the scar). This makes these muscles much more susceptible to injury.

Once this extremely common problem is detected, many have devised their own way to tone, strengthen and condition the muscles. Once accomplished, this partially injured muscle appears to be no more susceptible to injury than any other muscle.

Unfortunately, there hasn't been a good system that has helped everyone. Now with Opti-stretch, a good scientific system exists. It can document that the muscles are not completely healed. The "weak link" can be detected.

The asymptomatic chronically injured muscle not only constitutes the major risk factor for recurrent back pain, but also is something that can be eliminated through using the Opti-stretch therapeutic programs. Specific screening stretches give a very "reproducible measurement" of the amount of muscle tightness. A measurable degree of tightness from one side of the body compared to the other side is referred to as an abnormality in body symmetry. Detection of differences in body symmetry, due to asymptomatic chronically injured muscles (ACIMs), is the major goal of the Opti-stretch screening program. There are several other causes of differences in body symmetry, such as shortening of bone, tendons and ligaments. These other causes are usually not correctable to the extent that the asymptomatic chronically injured muscle can be corrected.

5. MUSCLE TONE

Opti-stretch therapeutic exercises are designed to restore muscle tone. Several definitions of muscle tone exist. The definition used in this book is the definition used by the general population. Recently this concept has been popularized to represent a normal state of flexibility and general health of the muscle. It is a muscle with optimum elasticity and range of motion.

Opti-stretch data suggests the range of motion for an individual is highly dependent on several factors. Age, gender, height, frame size, "double-jointedness" and muscle tone are important determinants. Constructing a normogram for the first 5 factors allows a predicted average range of motion for a given body type. Variance from predicted flexibility for specific body types provides an indication of muscle tone. The key to this data is the accurate, reproducible and a relatively easy determination of range of motion. Stretching exercises allow for this type of measurement.

Opti-stretch defines muscle tone as the distance stretched from the "first sensation of stretch" to where some level of discomfort is felt (either mild, moderate, or moderately severe). The more toned the muscle, the more intensity of force can be applied. Also, a greater stretch distance is achieved before a given level of discomfort is reached (such as moderate discomfort). In toned muscles, the levels of mild, moderate, moderately-severe, and severe discomfort are easily recognized. Each has a specific range for a give muscle. Any foreshortening of this range is an indication that something is wrong with the muscle.

Now, for the first time, an objective measurement of an individuals muscle tone can be performed accurately with only simple measuring devices (measuring tape and aneroid manometer). While large populations have not yet been studied, the accuracy of these parameters should allow certain comparisons between different size and type of muscles. Also, certain comparisons between specific body types may be available (see Graph 2, page 89). Of significant interest, both from a scientific and a clinical standpoint, is the early similarity and later differences for a poorly toned muscle (i.e., ACIM) and a healthy muscle. The early parts of both graphs are very similar for a measured small distance of stretch. The marked difference is in the later part of the graph. The healthy muscle will move relatively much further and withstand a much greater intensity of measured force in millimeters of mercury pressure. The healthy muscle usually has 4 discernible transition points from "stretch to pain". The poorly toned muscle or an ACIM typically has only 2 or 3 transition points. A severe acutely injured muscle will usually have only 1 transition point, which is about 8 to 10 millimeters or less of mercury pressure. By using the above Opti-stretch principles, muscle tone can be more scientifically defined and in the future help identify realistic parameters.

After the age of 35, accessory (secondary) stretch receptors can be demonstrated, before the muscle is warmed up. Once the muscle is warmed up, the individual will feel the primary stretch receptors of the muscles, just as the young do. They also can begin to feel the other stretch receptors in the musculo-skeletal system such as ligaments and tendons.

Excessive tone in core muscles does exist. In those that engage in certain sports that require extensive range of motion, excessive tone can be developed (acquired or environmental). This rarely presents a problem. However, there is a fairly large percentage of the population (10 to 20%) who will demonstrate some aspect of double-jointedness. This is considered a congenital condition and conveys to the individual a certain amount of extensive tone dependent on the degree of double-jointedness. Often, these double-jointed individuals will demonstrate a significantly different pattern of back reinjury compared with those individuals who are not double-jointed. Opti-stretch theory believes that because of the excessive tone, the muscles do not adequately protect other skeletal structures, which can then lead to muscle, joint and ligament injury.

Be aware that in the medical literature "tonus" or tone, when applied to muscles has a somewhat different and very specific scientific and medical definition. It generally applies to antigravity muscles. Both the lack of tone (hypotonicity) and too much tone (hypertonicity) of the muscles can be detected. Either of these two conditions can be associated with an increase in muscle strain.

6. Stretch Receptors

"Stretch receptors" is another term that varies between the medical community and the general public. Muscle stretch receptors have been specifically identified on a cellular basis and extensively studied in animals. Also, there exist specific stretch receptors of tendons that make the leg jump when tapped with a doctor's reflex hammer. Most of this physiology has been worked out in the animal model.

The process by which the above-mentioned receptors (and possibly other types of muscle receptors) produce the graded sensation of discomfort that human beings feel when a muscle is stretched, may actually be much more complex than previously thought. The subtleties of this particular phenomenon are difficult to experiment with in animals and even more difficult to experiment with in humans.

Opti-stretch studies suggest that there may be at least two or more separate stretch receptors, a primary and an accessory receptor. The accessory stretch receptor is usually not apparent during youth or in toned muscles. As the individual ages and tone starts to diminish, the influence of the accessory stretch receptor becomes more apparent.

Children are able to obtain an optimal stretch of their muscles at just about any time of the day. Individuals over 35 years of age often notice a sensation related to the accessory stretch receptor that is felt consistently at a certain distance of stretch. If the muscle is then warmed up, using various techniques, the muscle can be stretched further to the primary receptor level. Once the muscles are warmed up and stretched to the optimum, the accessory stretch receptor is then dormant until the muscles are immobile for at least two to three hours. After this immobility, the accessory stretch receptor is reset to precisely the original degree of limited stretch.

This helps to explain why, as one ages, the muscles seem to get stiff following a long plane or car ride. It also may explain why individuals, over the age of 35, may not see a significant change if practicing stretching routines that only engage the accessory stretch receptor. For this reason, a warm up phase is built into the Opti-stretch Therapeutic Technique.

One thing is clear; there are several different types of stretch receptor conditions. Opti-stretch is designed to help you differentiate between an acute injury stretch receptor, a chronic injury stretch receptor, an accessory receptor and a primary receptor. If an accessory stretch receptor exists, one can safely learn to work through to the primary receptor by warming up the muscle and thereby, helping to avoid injury of this more sensitive receptor. However, if one tries to work through a primary receptor, or an acute injury stretch receptor, the chance of significant injury to the muscle is extremely high.

7. INVOLUNTARY STRETCHING – (INSTINCTIVE STRETCHING)

Nature teaches us a great deal about stretch receptors and their importance. The word "stretching" originally referred to a very characteristic involuntary stretch reflex that every mammal demonstrates (with the exception of marine mammals). Presumably, marine mammals do not need to stretch because they never stop moving for prolonged periods from the time they are first born. They even swim in their sleep. Terrestrial mammals all have some type of prolonged inactivity (usually during sleep) and demonstrate an instinctive stretching routine upon awakening or getting up from a prolonged rest. In higher vertebrates, the most universal stretch is a bending of the lumbar spine backward (referred to as a backbend). Most everyone has seen a dog or other animal stretch. This is a genetically controlled involuntary reflex movement and referred to as an instinctive stretch in animals.

In some forms of vertebrates, such as ducks, very characteristic stretching routines are used for their wings even among different species. This also is genetically programmed and appears to be more of a stretching routine rather than a reflex type of movement observed in higher vertebrates.

Study of involuntary (instinctive) stretching in mammals may seem rather insignificant, but many important discoveries in medicine have been made while attempting to explain why certain phenomena exist in multiple species (the process of teleology). An expression used frequently in medicine and science is that "common things are common".

A classic involuntary stretch, in man, is the yawn. Certain muscles are relaxed while others are forcefully contracted to produce a very characteristic movement. Most of us know what it is like to yawn. It is something that can be imitated but not fully reproduced, through conscious effort. Furthermore, approaching the same range of motion of the jaw through conscious effort is quite uncomfortable. During an involuntary stretch, the involuntary portions of the brain can specifically relax certain muscles while contracting others. Most likely, there are many other complex physiologic processes responsible for a comfortable yawn.

Every healthy terrestrial mammal including man involuntarily stretches at birth. The onset is generally considered to be the "quickening" of the fetus. In most mammals this process continues until old age. The response then slowly decreases and finally stops altogether. Two things that will **stop** the instinctive stretching process in mammals for short periods are disease and injury. In the case of significant injury, the limb is held immobile by the animal. As the limb starts healing, the mammal will start progressively moving and testing the movement of the limb. This progresses to gradual weight bearing and eventual complete return of movement to the limb. Once the limb has returned to near normal function, the instinctive stretching resumes. Dogs with an amputated front leg will resume instinctive stretching once the surgical incision has healed sufficiently.

The exact purpose of this involuntary stretch in terrestrial mammals is not well understood. One plausible theory is that it tones muscles and helps protect them from injury.

Following prolonged inactivity or sleep, involuntary stretch re-tones the muscles, making them less susceptible to injury. However, when a mammal is frightened from sleep, a phenomenon referred to as the "fight or flight response" occurs. In this case adrenaline immediately re-tones the muscles and powerfully maximizes immediate muscular performance, while at the same time decreasing the chance of muscular injury.

One explanation, as to why the instinctive stretching usually stops at old age, is that this type of stretching may be extremely important for maintaining the muscular health of individual members of a species. In nature "survival of the fittest" is an essential principle. Many known genetically programmed physiological phenomena exist that help animals to survive in the reproductive years. However, beyond this point and into old age, there are other types of programmed physiological phenomena that actually help the animal pass through old age as quickly as possible. The cessation of stretching is seen in old age, as well as, during significant disease and injury. Therefore, in theory, continuing to do stretching, as one ages, might actually help slow the aging process and preserve muscular vitality for years longer. For those that have lost muscular vitality and tone through lack of activity or chronic injury, regaining this muscular health can be like discovering a "fountain of youth".

Humans are quite unique as a species in that only a minority of individuals continue to demonstrate instinctive or involuntary stretching past the time of puberty. The number of individuals who do not perform involuntary stretches appear to be more common in Western societies and other "modern" societies. This may well be due to the stresses and hectic lifestyles commonly seen in these societies. It may be as simple as a lack of activity with specific range of motion, which can lead to detoning of the muscles and subsequent cessation of the involuntary stretch. However, extensive research has not yet been done in this area.

Healthy individuals (many who work on farms) report this type of involuntary stretching even at ages 60 to 70. Opti-stretch has demonstrated that once the muscles are optimally toned, the involuntary stretching can return, even following decades of cessation.

Stretching exercises, first popularized in Western cultures during the 1940's, are purported to tone muscles and help slow the natural aging process. Using an extension of the argument expressed above, the most important muscles to be stretched would be those muscles involved with involuntary stretching. The most important muscles stretched with an involuntary stretch are the core muscles of the body. Furthermore, like the yawn, gaining the same level of range of motion as generated by the subconscious mind in an involuntary stretch is very difficult by implementing general stretching exercise techniques commonly in practice today. The most popular technique of stretching is to stretch to a level of mild or moderate discomfort and hold for 30 seconds. If one opens the mouth to simulate a yawn only to the level of mild discomfort and holds for 30 seconds, the range of motion is significantly less than the range of motion generated with a normal involuntary yawn. You will note that attempting to imitate the range of motion of the yawn will result in moderately-severe discomfort. From experience, we know that if one pushes the discomfort level to severe discomfort or to the level of actual pain, acute strain injury of the muscle can occur. All these and many more factors have been investigated by Opti-stretch in order to have an effective but injury safe program.

A stretching exercise does not just stretch a single muscle. However, for any given stretch one certain muscle or group of muscles receives the maximum amount of stress generated during that stretch. By consistently coupling the fixed position of other joints, certain muscles can be more specifically isolated. This is why there can be multiple stretching positions designed to stretch even a single muscle. As previously suggested above, instinctive stretches may have more physiological significance than previously recognized. In watching many children and infants stretch, there appear to be many similarities just as there are many similarities when individuals yawn.

The most commonly observed pattern of involuntary stretching in humans involves pulling the shoulder blades closer together and bending the spine backwards at the level of the low back (or backbend). In this position, the psoas muscle receives the most stress of all the low back muscles. The psoas muscle is one of the most complex muscles of the body. It will be explained in more detail later (see Section 14. The Psoas Muscle). Furthermore, it is important to note that the different patterns and type of movement generated by involuntary stretching are not common movements in most routine daily activities in humans, especially in Western culture.

During the above involuntary stretch, the upper back and arm stretches are equally interesting. Individuals, who still experience involuntary stretching, describe a significant sensation of muscle well-being in-between the shoulder blades. Only a small stretch is perceived in the front part of the shoulders. However, between the shoulder blades, the rhomboid muscles are actually contracting and not stretching. This is because the rhomboids are one of the few muscles that are very difficult to stretch due to the function of the shoulder and shoulder blade (scapula). If one tries to perform a stretching exercise for the shoulder blades, the rhomboids are protected from stretch by other more sensitive shoulder muscles. One of the best ways to tone and condition the rhomboid muscles is to maximally contract the muscles rather than stretching them. Mother Nature may have guessed that the average human was not going to stumble on to this concept too easily, so she programmed it into an involuntary stretch for humans. From a teleological standpoint, the precise reasons for involuntary stretching are quite intriguing.

In summary, the classic involuntary stretch seen in all healthy infants involves arm, upper back and lower back movement. Stretching of the arms and upper back seems to be centered on the area between the shoulder blades (specifically the greater and lesser rhomboid muscles). The simultaneous stretch of the low back appears to center around the psoas muscle complex.

8. Range of Motion

In medicine, range of motion is the distance a given joint will move by the muscles powering that joint for a specific plane of motion. Many comprehensive Orthopedic textbooks have multiple pages of normal values for the range of motion of any given joint. "Stretched range of motion" is a valuable tool for physical therapists. It is a technique commonly used to regain normal joint range of motion. Seldom is it routinely measured and reported in textbooks. In part, this is because the variability is so large within a given population. However, Opti-stretch has found that if double-jointed individuals are placed in a separate group, the stretched range of motion is quite uniform given age, gender, height, and frame size. If an optimum stretched range of motion can be predicted for a given individual, then the measured "stretched range of motion" would be directly proportional to muscle tone and indirectly proportional to tight muscles (given normal healthy joints, ligaments and tendons).

Traditionally, joint motion is measured in the frontal plane and sagital plane (two separate planes). This is the best way of simplifying the body's complex movement capabilities. Hip and shoulder joints are able to undergo significant rotation. Assuming up to 360 degrees in one-degree increments, this would make the flexion and extension slightly different in at least 360 different planes. In actuality, the body is infinitely more complex and fractions of a degree can make a huge difference in the movement of a joint. Not only are many joints able to undergo hundreds of different planes of movement, but the movement of one joint is effected by the position of other joints, usually in proximity to the joint. This allows significant coupling of a joint's motion relative to the position of another joint.

The easiest way to both describe and measure these complex couplings of joints is to fix the given limb and the opposite limb as much as possible. The one limb is then moved through a simple standard plane of motion. One very simple example is to extend the fingers and the thumb of one hand. Then touch the tip of the thumb to the palm of the hand, just below the little finger. Try to extend the fingers of the hand. The index and middle finger become difficult to fully extend.

Traditionally, range of motion is measured in degrees of flexion, extension or rotation of the joint. A goniometer is a device that measures this angle. It takes a very skilled anatomist to generate any type of reproducible measurement when multiple joints (especially those of the spine) are involved. This suggests that a skilled anatomist needs to be present, or a photograph generated, each time the individual wants to obtain feedback regarding his or her improvement in stretching distance. By coupling the joints consistently and standardizing the position each time, the individual has excellent reproducible feedback as to the progress. These motions also closely simulate the complex movements the joints and muscles are normally called upon in order to perform certain more strenuous activities.

To simplify the measuring technique even further, the movement is measured by the distance between two given objects (such as the nose and knee). Unfortunately, this data measured in inches cannot be accurately compared to other individuals, especially with different body types. Therefore, if you go to a medical textbook you will see range of motion only measured in degrees of the given angle of motion. While the Opti-stretch method of measurement is not as scientifically acceptable, it does provide extremely valuable and useful data to the individual. It also gives a measurement by which certain general but not exact comparisons can be made between individuals (i.e., some people have longer necks or noses).

Coupling joint motion is not a new concept. In fact, the concept has been used in certain martial arts for thousands of years. However, this type of application used by Opti-stretch is not commonly utilized, partially due to its somewhat inferior scientific value. In my opinion, the value to the individual and to his or her personal trainer is well worth it.

An example, is the "Sitting Nose to Knee" stretching exercise – (Figure Four). One of the muscles in question (the psoas muscle) travels over eight separate joints. In addition, movements of the vertebral facet joints are extremely difficult to measure with a goniometer. The individual range of motion of 14 separate joints would have to be measured individually to generate completely accurate scientific data for this one stretch alone. It would take over 30 minutes to perform the precise measurements. In addition, accurate measurements of subtle rotations of the spinal vertebrae are extremely difficult, even with x-ray. The bottom line is that using the Opti-stretch techniques of specific joint fixation, a simplified process of measuring certain complex movements can be achieved, which is both accurate and reproducible for a given individual.

9. Hyperflexibility and Double-jointedness

Literally, hyperflexibility implies greater flexibility than the average individual. Hyperflexibility is also a term often used to describe double-jointed individuals. Double-jointed individuals (who actually demonstrate true joint hyperextensibility) do tend to be more flexible.

To extend the arm, you simply straighten your arm. A double-jointed individual not only can straighten the arm out, but they can bend it backwards a little ways.

If all forms of double-jointedness are considered, including thumb hyperextensibility, the condition is extremely common. Roughly 10 to 20 percent of the population have some measurable hyperextensibility of at least one joint. This suggests that between 10 and 20 percent of the population have some degree of genetic hyperflexibility . This is usually seen more often in females.

Remember, this 20 percent of the population are not same 20 percent in the "never any back pain" group. As mentioned earlier, for centuries it has been known that the more flexible the individual, does not necessarily mean the less back problems the individual will have. In fact, hyperflexible individuals often suffer very significantly from recurrent back strain problems.

In order to help this group of hyperflexible individuals, it is important to first be able to recognize the group. For simplicity, Opti-stretch has utilized a very basic screening process than can identify individuals who display some amount of genetic hyperextensibility. Opti-stretch simply looks for small, medium and large joint hyperextensibility. The larger the joint which is hyperextensible, the more the general amount of hyperflexibility that is seen between ages 6 and 45. Over age 55 there appears to be less of a correlation. Many senior citizens with demonstrable joint hyperextensibility actually tend to be similar or even less flexible than the general population.

Below, are listed the four degrees of genetic hyperextensibility. Also listed are the corresponding joints (examined during the Opti-stretch research). There is a noticeable difference in general flexibility of the body between "normal" and each of the groups of one through fourth degree hyperextensibility (during childhood and young adulthood).

1° **Thumb:** Gently try to touch the thumb to the forearm as seen in Figure 4. This figure demonstrates the normal range of motion of the thumb. If you can touch the thumb to the forearm or even within the width of one finger from the forearm, you are considered to have first degree or small joint hyperflexibility.

FIGURE 4 – NORMAL THUMB RANGE OF MOTION

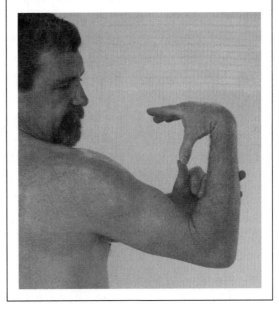

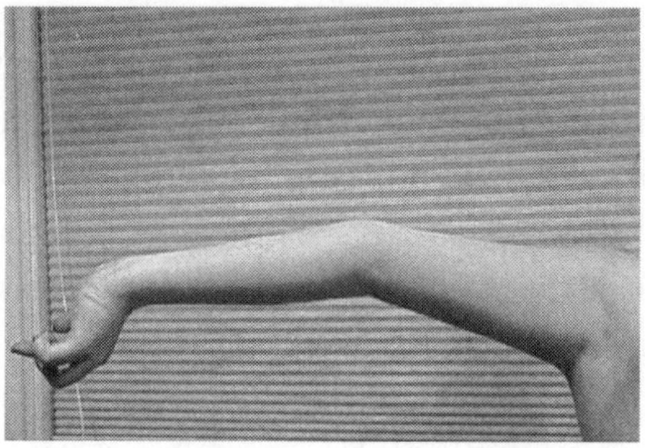

2° **Elbow:** If you can hyperextend the arm, you are considered to have second degree or medium joint hyperflexibility. Note in Figure 5, how the forearm can be bent backwards.

3° **Knee:** If you can hyperextend the knee you are considered to have third degree or large joint hyperflexibility. This is simply bending the knee backwards.

FIGURE 5 – HYPERFLEXIBILITY – ELBOW RANGE OF MOTION

4° **Back:** Significant hyperextension of the back. Usually only assessed in the individual who can perform the "Bridge" exercise. If the feet can be brought over the shoulders, this more extreme condition is commonly referred to as contortion. This is a rare condition. However, mild and moderate hyperextension of the back is quite common.

Anyone, with other than first-degree hyperextensibility, needs to be aware that some of the Opti-stretch exercises like (Figure Four) and (Butterfly) may be accomplished without difficulty. This makes these two very important learning stretches not very useful. However, in working with several hyperextensible individuals with either acute back pain or recurrent injury, an asymmetry was found in these two stretching exercises. They were unable to touch the nose to the knee on the side where they had back pain. Therefore, it is advisable to use the program as it currently exists, until a better one can be devised for the hyperextensible groups.

A very common pattern of injury in this group is due to the combination of hyperflexibility and joint hyperextensibility. Joints appear to be less protected by stretch receptor reflexes. Joint and ligament trauma then causes indirect muscle spasm and associated back pain.

10. PROPRIOCEPTIVE NEUROMUSCULAR FACILITATION (PLF)

The concept of proprioceptive neuromuscular facilitation (PLF) is important to mention. It is one of the more effective ways to stretch a muscle and to achieve stretch receptor lengthening of a muscle. It is frequently used when working with certain trainers and health care professionals. Basically, the trainer stretches a muscle until there is a mild to moderate stretch on the muscle. At that point, the individual being stretched contracts the muscle against a fixed resistance of the trainer, in an isometric fashion. As the muscle starts to fatigue, the muscle is then relaxed and slightly more force is placed by the trainer in order to stretch it further. The process is repeated until a moderate to moderately severe stretch is placed on the muscle. Certified personal trainers and licensed health care professionals should be the only ones doing this on another person.

However, an individual performing stretches can use a similar technique. The resistance is simply a force applied by the arms helping to perform and control the stretch.

PLF is not recommended at near maximum stretch. It is far too difficult to think about the amount of stress provided by the arms and then trying to think about a contracting force in the leg muscle. You need all your concentration on finding precisely the maximum end point. The risk of injury is too great by using PLF at near maximum stretch. However, it can be an effective warm-up technique if you are already familiar with it.

As mentioned above, it is not necessary to know or use the PLF technique with Opti-stretch. **Warning; do <u>not</u> use PLF on the "Sitting Nose to Knee" – (Figure Four).**

What happens is that an injury will occur to the psoas muscle on the opposite leg. To hold resistance for isometric contractions takes approximately 50 pounds of force for an average male. The same mechanics and forces would be analogous to standing on a step and keeping the left leg straight, to simulate stretching the left leg. Next, the individual would have to bend the right leg and place the foot on a one-foot high cinderblock. Next, if someone were foolish enough to reach down and pick up a 50-pound weight below the level of the left foot, this would place the same force on the right psoas muscle, as would the (Figure Four) exercise using PLF. The right psoas has to stabilize the back. A significant muscle strain of the right psoas is almost guaranteed, due to the twisting angle of the right psoas muscle used to stabilize the back in this position.

Again, do not use PLF with (Figure Four). Nor is it advisable to use this with any other Opti-stretch stretching exercise, unless you know precisely what you are doing. It simply isn't worth the risk.

11. ACUTE MUSCLE INJURY

How do you know the difference between an acute muscle injury, reinjury pattern or a chronic muscle injury? This unfortunately is a difficult concept to teach but it can be learned by experience.

Acute injury means there has been some type of acute tissue damage. The skin, bones, ligaments and muscles all heal at about the same rate for a severe injury. Often minor injuries are much more subtle and difficult to detect. For example, you may feel fine on a given day. However, by chance you may touch a spot on your skin that is tender. If there is no bruise, most likely you will remember bumping the area a day or two prior. However, if it not only feels tender and you can see a bruise, you will recall the event that caused this injury. Often the black-and-blue skin changes may take a few days to form and confirm your suspicions.

A skin bruise is simply skin that received sufficient stress and damage, which was sufficient to break tiny blood vessels. All healthy tissues are the same. A muscle bruise and a bone bruise have roughly the same amount of blood that has leaked from tiny blood vessels for a given mild injury. However, frequently you can't see or medically confirm this problem other than touching the area for tenderness. A bruise and a strain will heal exactly the same way (over time).

Most everyone has strained an ankle or other joint. There is almost always a sensation of something "not being right". If it is very mild, you may still continue running on the ankle. However, by the end of the day, the ankle may be swollen and painful. Then, you are certain you have at least sprained the ankle. Remember the only medical difference between a strain and a sprain is that you or your doctor can identify traumatic changes like swelling or skin bruising with a sprain. If you only strain the ankle, no differences may be clinically seen. However, the ankle still hurts when you try to move or bear weight on it. There are many joints, like the ankle, that can appear only to have sustained a strain. However, on x-ray evaluation a small piece of bone may have been broken off. Even if it is only a small bone chip, this is still considered to be a severely sprained ankle and usually requires several weeks of healing. If a cast or walking splint is not applied, the usual way to heal the ankle is to apply an ace wrap and limp around for a few days. Eventually, as the swelling and pain decrease, the limp decreases also. Gradually, more activity then can be applied to the ankle. During this later stage of healing of an acute ankle strain or sprain, stretching exercises can be of value.

However, it you sustained a badly sprained ankle and started stretching exercises that same day and each day following, chances are you would actually slow the healing process. This is because there would be a prolongation of the inflammatory phase of healing. You would be subjecting yourself to needless discomfort. As mentioned earlier, there are some tissues that will never heal properly if you continue to irritate them and fail to let nature heal the tissue to at least a certain level.

A small skin cut that forms a scab is the classic example. If the scab is removed every day so there is even a little bit of bleeding, that skin lesion will never heal in the lifetime of the individual. The broken bone, if moved daily, will often abnormally heal in 2 pieces instead of one. During severe injuries like a broken bone, the body, in order to protect and promote healing, causes severe spasm to all agonistic, accessory and antagonistic muscles of that area. This effectively immobilizes the bone fragments to promote healing. Also, intense pain results with any type of motion, effectively preventing motion until the bone or injury has sufficiently healed. In modern medicine, a cast is usually applied to both immobilize and decrease the reflex muscle spasm.

Severely strained muscles and ligaments sometimes heal better with a cast. However, the majority of the time mild and moderate strains usually heal better without a cast. Medical doctors will usually provide a splint, sling, crutch, or guidelines for use, to provide enough protection to where the injury will start to heal. As it feels better, you are instructed to gently increase mobility and use, until the area returns to normal. However, if the injury does not return to normal or if the injury remains too painful for too long, you are instructed to return for further evaluation. Too painful and too long are both something you have to judge by experience, while the medical doctor learns these parameters through training.

Many individuals, who are experiencing a severe strain injury for the first time in the extremities, will return to a doctor after a couple of weeks thinking a bone is broken. An X-ray with bone spicule formation within the strained muscle will definitively demonstrate that the strain was indeed severe. The patient is reassured that another four to six weeks may be necessary for complete healing. However, they are usually instructed to return if it has not healed by at least two months. Very few severe injuries take longer than two months to significantly improve. More importantly, if there has been a complication in the healing process and if the individual waits much longer than two months, the complication may have healed to a point where it is not easily treated. Most people learn about these things either through four years of medical school, personal experience as an overactive kid, or "Dr. Mom."

Injuries to the muscles of the back are no exception. If you try stretching the muscles before they have had a chance to heal to at least a certain point, you are probably wasting your time and possibly prolonging the inflammation phase of the injury.

One notable exception is the stiff and sore muscle. When overuse of a muscle leads to stiffness and soreness the next day, gentle stretching exercises can be very helpful in clearing the lactic acid build up more rapidly. When the muscle is acutely stiff and sore, it is significantly more susceptible to injury. However, if the lactic acid is cleared by an hour or two of movement, usually a near maximum performance of the muscle can be expected without any significant risk of injury.

So how do you differentiate between a minimally injured (stiff and sore) muscle and a mildly injured muscle? This is not an easy question to answer. Often stiff and sore muscles are actually more painful and incapacitating than a mild or moderately injured muscle. As a general rule of thumb, stiff and sore muscles usually involve multiple muscles. A strain involves usually only one muscle, except when it is a moderate strain and involves the agonistic and accessory muscles. In a severe strain, three different muscle groups are often involved (agonistic, accessory, and antagonistic). This concept is discussed more fully under the topic Chiropractic and Other Manipulations in Section 18.

Detecting, acute strains and properly dealing with them, is something that can be learned with time and experience. When you originally learn the Opti-stretch technique, it is by comparing healthy muscles to asymptomatic chronically injured muscles (ACIMs). The individual then may feel great for months. Then one day he or she overdoes it or performs an activity they are not used to. <u>Mild</u> acute muscle injuries often feel very similar to an asymptomatic chronically injured muscle. Therefore, they attempt to continue using Opti-stretch techniques and either don't get the same relief or actually make the mild acutely-strained condition worse. This is an extremely common mistake. Because individuals are taught in the Opti-stretch technique to be aware of distances for the purpose of positive feedback and effective measurement of progress, many often mistakenly try to stretch to a given distance rather than a given sensation.

The concept of "Oh, I'll just try a little harder to reach that distance" is very dangerous and is completely against what Opti-stretch tries to teach. The concept that needs to be adhered to is referred to as the "just right" or "the Goldielocks" phenomenon. <u>**More is not better**</u>. Too cold or too little, may not be enough. However, too hot or too much may be injurious. "Just right" is a concept that varies among people and must be learned individually.

Remember that a stiff and sore muscle will be effectively worked out in one to two hours by using gentle warm-up exercises. If the soreness persists longer, it usually indicates a mild injury. The mild injury will tend to get worse or not be improved after the two hour maximum. Sometimes after an extremely strenuous day of say digging ditches, it takes one to two hours to effectively work out the stiffness and soreness on awakening. A second hard day's work can then be safely performed. However, if I am able to work out only part of the stiffness and soreness using 80% MAX (moderate discomfort), I may return the following day to digging ditches but I will try to be a lot more careful and cautious for a day or two, in order to avoid a muscle strain. The same thing applies to play.

If I'm up on a beautiful mountain for a day of skiing and find I'm a little stiff and sore from the ride up or from the day before, I don't turn around and go home. I just perform the stretches to a level that I comfortably can. This level is no more than 80% MAX [moderate discomfort] for any minimal or mild injury. If I cannot reach my normal level of stretch, I don't just try harder or exceed the moderate discomfort level. If, I'm a few inches off my normal level, I simply use a little more caution and avoid extreme skiing for at least the morning. After lunch, I reassess the muscles to determine how aggressive I can be for the rest of the day.

However, if I determine that there is an acute <u>moderate</u> injury to a muscle, I will spend the day in the lodge rather than risk the chance of a severe injury. These concepts are very basic. While this knowledge is usually learned by trial and error by individuals, Opti-stretch can be of significant value in providing a more objective assessment of the possibility that an acute injury has occurred.

To make things more complex, you may not even realize you have a mild or moderate injury until you move the muscle. You may not even know you have injured a muscle until you are doing your Opti-stretch stretching exercises the following day. That is why you always perform a detection (Check and Stretch) and then a gentle warm up (mild discomfort) to detect any hidden abnormalities. If you are not performing warm up exercises before attempting 80% MAX stretches, you are not doing the Opti-stretch technique properly. You may erroneously conclude that the stretch you are doing that morning injured the muscle. While this could be possible, more commonly you will be able to recall some unusual activity with that area of the body from the day before. If you do not warm up the muscles properly before attempting a moderate discomfort intensity level, you can very easily convert a mild strain into a moderate strain.

In either of the three cases above, you have, by definition, sustained an <u>acute muscle injury</u>. Stop stretching for at least two days, apply ice, and try to protect the area from overuse. Then start carefully resuming the exercises after at least two days rest and only at mild discomfort (50% MAX) intensity. Over the next few days, gradually work up your intensity level if you are feeling better.

Moderate or severe injuries are a little more straight forward. Usually, you will have at least some sensation that the muscle has been pulled or injured. It may take two to eight hours before a more severe pain begins to set in. This is why I have included the following classification of normal healing processes (see next page, <u>Table 2</u>). By simply judging the amount of pain, you may not be able to determine precisely the extent of an injury. However, by measuring the length of time it takes to heal a muscle given optimum care, you can retroactively assess more accurately how badly the muscle was injured. This system works well, because we are usually dealing with reoccurring strains and **Opti-stretch is not designed for acute injuries.**

TABLE 2 – ACUTE MUSCLE INJURY

1. __Minimal injury.__ This consists of stiff and sore muscles that can generally be worked out in at least two hours by no more than 80% MAX (moderate discomfort). If they cannot, then you have, by definition, a mild injury.

2. __Mild injury.__ This injury is associated with mild pain on movement of the muscle. It will usually return to essentially normal in two to three days. If I think I have a mild injury, I stop stretching for two days, apply ice for 20 minutes at least once a day, and try to avoid as much activity to that area as possible, so as to rest and heal the muscle.

3. __Moderate injury.__ This injury is associated with moderate pain and usually remains painful at rest. I don't even bother to try stretching these muscles. Ice therapy with the application of ice for 20 minute every one to two hours for at least the first couple of days is recommended. In five to seven days the pain at rest noticeably subsides. Gentle stretching can then be attempted. Start at 50% MAX intensity. This injury usually heals back to normal in about one to two weeks.

4. __Severe injury.__ These injuries always produce some sensation of injury immediately at the time of occurrence. However, on occasion the severe pain may not start for two to eight hours. It often will gradually build up in intensity. Severe pain is defined by an inability to walk comfortably or find a comfortable place to rest, even while lying down. Simple activities like putting on your shoes may take 20 minutes. In speaking with hundreds of individuals who have suffered severe muscle strain, they rank it among their most intensely painful experiences in life both due to intensity of pain and length of healing. The pain ranks right up there with broken bones, heart attacks, and major operations. A physician should always evaluate this type of severe pain. William's Flexion Exercises are the gold standard for acute care of a severely strained back. These usually can be started safely after a few days or the first week. However, Opti-stretch techniques should not be attempted until you can rest comfortably in bed and can walk fairly normally. This is generally at least two to four weeks. Always restart with the Beginning Exercises. Never exceed 50% MAX for the first two months or until your physician officially states it is all right. You need to be cleared for regular activity.

Opti-stretch puts significant stress on the lumbar core muscles and hence, on the lumbar discs. Instead of a severe muscle strain, it is possible that you could have just as easily sustained a partially herniated disc. Although it has not yet happened, in theory, it could be possible to convert a small herniated disc into a major herniated disc requiring back surgery. Don't attempt anything above 50% MAX exercises for at least two months or until your Orthopedic Surgeon has released you to normal activity. If you don't know where your 50% MAX level is for sure, __don't do Opti-stretch__ until released by a physician for normal activity or at least six months of healing has occurred.

Opti-stretch, so far, has proven much like other forms of therapy for acute injury. It may make you feel a little better sooner, by taking out some of the spasm, but it simply does not heal an acute injury faster. Once the injury has healed sufficiently, __then__ Opti-stretch may be extremely useful in regaining 100% health to the muscle. But remember; do not employ this therapy until the muscle is properly healed.

Don't try to push any acute injury! Don't even push stiff and sore muscles! The Opti-stretch technique is very powerful and therefore, very dangerous in acute muscle injuries and injuries that involve the fascia or bones. You will also be happy to know that any progress you have made in your range of motion usually does not significant-ly change for about one to three weeks. The bottom line is that if you don't know where things are with healing or if you are not steadily improving, simply **avoid all Opti-stretch activities** for at least two months after a severe injury, or until you have received a formal medical consultation. This is especially important **whenever** you suspect any acute injury that is not progressing along the time frames given above.

12. WARMING UP

The muscles are maximally protected during the fight-or-flight response. In an emer-gency situation adrenaline is released. This chemical is known to provide maximum performance of the muscles while decreasing the chance of muscle injury. In non-emergency situations where adrenaline is not produced, a warm up is essential to pre-vent injury to muscles. This is especially important as one ages.

Remember stretching routines are just one of many types of warm-up routines. Warm-up routines vary significantly from sport to sport and from individual to individual. The most effective routine is one that works for the individual and is practiced on a reg-ular basis.

Professional basketball players have a definite warm-up routine. It involves gradually increasing in intensity the movements that will be required at the opening tip off. First, there is a period of shooting the basketball with sweats on. When they feel completely warmed up, the sweats come off and a few complex moves are tried before the start of the game. (Note that when the player is warming up an injured leg or ankle, the routine is markedly different.) This type of routine works well for many athletes and many sports.

In contrast, the college and professional football players have a very elaborate warm-up routine, which includes stretches and calisthenics. Then some jumping and bouncing techniques are implemented prior to running a few 1/2 speed plays. For sports where the body can be forced into multiple positions at the very start of the game, each and every muscle must be warmed up.

The above two types of warm ups are both excellent for the given sport. The main con-cept is that unless the muscles are warmed up, there is a much greater possibility of injury. I am amazed at many young athletes who have a warm-up routine for their school sports or recreational softball team. They would never dream of playing an intercollegiate game of football or race at a track meet without warming-up. However, when it comes to a day of skiing or a hard day of manual labor, they often never even think about warming-up the muscles.

Opti-stretch stretching exercises really should be looked upon as a sport when the intensity levels reach a moderate or moderately-severe level of discomfort. The muscles have to be warmed up or the chance of injury is higher. While stretching exercises are the very best way for checking for partially injured muscles and checking for range of motion, they serve as only a part of a good total warm-up process.

I like to compare and experiment with various warm-up techniques before proceeding to stretch receptor lengthening. Many different warm-up techniques can be found in almost any book on exercising. This is an excellent way of comparing a specific warm-up technique with those of the Opti-stretch set. It is nice to have two or three different types of warm-up techniques depending on the activity you want to engage in. One technique is utilized when there is only a short warm-up period. Another technique may be used as an optimum warm-up method for the start of a very intense activity. Still others might need to be used to avoid fatiguing the muscles when immediate maximum strength exertion of the muscles is required, as in a sprint or race. Stretching, too long (over three minutes per muscle) or too hard, can fatigue muscles. This may be a factor in some Olympic sprinters no longer performing stretching exercises immediately before a race.

Muscles can be significantly fatigued at the moderate and higher discomfort level of stretch. This is one of the reasons why at these levels, Opti-stretch sets are recommended for only two to three sets per workout session. Avoiding fatigue is important in reducing the chance of injury. This is also why high levels of stretch intensity should be avoided prior to certain athletic sports event.

Considering time efficiency and effectiveness together, the Opti-stretch warm-up technique is the best I have found for the main core muscles of the body. Each of the Opti-stretch stretching exercises isolates specific core muscles. Once these core muscles are properly warmed up, the peripheral muscles are usually ready to go (unless there is a specific problem or injury to a peripheral muscle). In extreme activities, calisthenics are often performed to test for and ensure peripheral muscle warm up.

The bottom line is that stretching exercises are only one type of warm-up technique. Other warm-up techniques are just as effective in warming up certain muscles prior to activities. However, for warming up muscles, checking for injury and assessing optimum range of motion for a given activity, stretching exercises are extremely effective. Also, warming up the muscles is imperative prior to proceeding on to stretch receptor lengthening techniques.

In properly cooling down fatigued muscles, warm-up exercises have been shown to be extremely effective in preventing lactic acid build up. This helps prevent stiffness and soreness the following day after overexerting muscles.

13. THE PSOAS SHORT LEG SYNDROME

In the late 1800's, the first documentation of widespread leg shortening in the general public was published. Research documented that in over 50% of the population in various sample populations, there were individuals with one leg shorter than the other. British <u>military physicians</u> investigated this concept of a shorter leg and the association with a higher incidence of back pain, during the 1960's (Nichols, P.J.R., British Medical Journal, 1960, 1, 1863). Published in the British Medical Journal, the article was titled the "Short Leg Syndrome". It described an increased incidence of low back pain in 1000 British soldiers with one leg shorter than the other. Several other articles dealt with the correlation of back pain and unilateral leg shortening. Most of the data and articles dealing with the short leg syndrome came from England and never gained much popularity in the American medical community. However, this concept did gain a degree of popularity in the American general public because many sufferers of recurrent back pain knew they had one leg, which was shorter than the other.

Another group of British physicians then evaluated soldiers with a device called a "locating jig" and concluded "chronic back pain is thus unlikely to be part of the short leg syndrome". (Lancet, 1984 Aug 4, 2:8397, 256-8.) Opti-stretch research suggests that the "locating jig" only demonstrated that the majority of individuals with an observable clinical shortening of one leg did <u>not</u> have bone length differences. This suggests that the original <u>military physicians</u> were dealing with some type of functional shortening of one leg. Although, this subject has been referred to by various authors, no further scientific research on a "Short Leg Syndrome" has been conducted since that time. It is unfortunate that there have been no definitive large population studies with good control groups to either prove or disprove the theory of back pain associated with one shorter leg. Opti-stretch theory agrees with and supports the published findings of the British military physicians. Careful review of this original literature was extremely helpful in leading to some of the new scientific discoveries by Opti-stretch.

The father of modern Pain Management in the USA, Dr. John Bonica, championed the belief that a short leg might be associated with severe recurrent back pain. His early career in professional wrestling left him with severe recurrent back pain and he did have one leg that was shorter than the other. He was one of the only American physicians that publicly even recognized the possibility of a "short-leg syndrome".

Part of the lack of interest in this concept by the American medical community might have been due to the fact that chiropractors have focused on the leg length differences in back pain for at least the last 50 to 100 years. There have even been claims of being able to correct some types of leg length shortening. Patients with a leg length disparity, which could not be corrected, were sold lifts. Lifts are a heal insole placed in the shoe to compensate for the shortening of one leg.

Since the late 1980's, Orthopedic surgeons have taken a very conservative approach to the problem of one leg being shorter than the other and a general tendency not to prescribe lifts. Statistically, at least one in every 100 individuals has a measurable leg shorter than the other due to <u>bone length</u> differences. This shortness has been correlated with multiple standard measurement techniques and x-ray confirmation. Provided the difference is less than one inch, many of these individuals have no problem with either posture or back pain. Opti-stretch research concurs with this data.

In the 1970's and 1980's, a lift in one shoe was frequently recommended for a shorter leg by many types of physicians. Orthopedic surgeons noted several problems that occurred in the feet and ankles due to chronic lift use. Today, insole lifts, on only one side, are recommended much less frequently than in the past.

Opti-stretch research suggests that use of such a lift can help decrease some forms of back pain in the acute phase. However, chronic use of such a lift in an active individual can have <u>many</u> negative side effects. If you are going to consider a lift, it is recommended that an orthopedic surgeon be consulted.

Three separate causes have been published for the unilateral leg shortening (anatomical, maximal acute spasm and functional) of one leg. The most obvious is that the bone lengths are different for some reason (<u>anatomical shortened leg</u>). This occurs quite frequently in approximately 1% of the population. Often, this is considered a congenital condition. However, it can also occur with severe trauma to the growth portion of the bone (growth plate) prior to adulthood. Significant trauma to this area can prematurely halt future bone growth.

Orthopedic surgeons have reported up to a 2-inch shortening of the leg during "<u>maximum psoas spasm</u>". The exact mechanism as to how the leg shortens has not been completely described in the literature. Severe acute maximum spasm of the psoas muscle is quite rare. One medical condition that can cause this maximal spasm is due to a psoas abscess. The shortening resolves when the spasm heals.

In addition to an anatomical short leg, there also exists a "<u>functional</u> short leg". This is a shortening of the leg without any difference in respective bone lengths. This concept is superficially described in several medical textbooks as a probable contraction of the hip and back muscles, which can cause a shortening of the leg. This terminology has gained popularity in the literature since the 1990's. While the terminology is used, it is not precisely defined nor are there any generally accepted theories as to the cause of the pathophysiology. Even though this phenomenon has been described, no in-depth research has yet been conducted as to the exact muscles involved and how the condition is best treated. The leg length difference reported is usually quite subtle (often a 1/4 inch or less). The exact etiology is still in question but deals with hip and leg rotation causing a functional shortening of one leg and a resultant pelvic tilt.

A new fourth cause of leg length discrepancy has been documented by Opti-stretch research. It has been coined as a "variable psoas pathology". The majority of the Opti-stretch research has focused around this phenomenon. While this is, more than likely, a variant of a "functional short leg", it is placed in a separate category for two reasons. First, it often exceeds the 1/4 inch described in some medical texts. The second reason is that it has been documented to be able to change length. Primarily, it is believed to be due to a chronic partial spasm of the psoas muscle complex. When partial spasm is reversed, there can be a residual psoas tendon shortening of less than 1/4 inch. It has not been determined whether the prolonged spasm caused the tendon shortening, or whether the tendon shortening occurred genetically making the psoas muscle more susceptible to strain injury. Tendon shortening alone may behave similarly to the "functional short leg" as described in the medical literature and not necessarily contribute to any back pain.

Opti-stretch research suggests that during psoas spasm, the hip joint undergoes a very complex external twisting rotation that can leave the leg shortened at the hip joint. This most commonly results in a posterior rotation of the pelvis on that side. (However, anterior rotation of the pelvis is occasionally seen.) The pelvis on the shortened side then tilts downward, due to pelvic leveling. With certain specific measuring techniques, the leg functionally and clinically can be shortened 1/2 to even 1 full inch. Certain coupled stretching positions like the "Standing Squat," will show the shorter leg to be consistently more externally rotated. At this level of chronic muscle spasm, these individuals have an extremely high incidence of low back pain and frequently will demonstrate a recurrent back strain syndrome. Indeed, Opti-stretch research has shown that the majority of individuals with all of the various "recurrent back strain syndromes" have this "variable psoas pathology".

There appears to be various "recurrent back strain syndromes", which can involve either the neck, upper back or the lower back. The most common for the lower back is the "Psoas Short Leg Syndrome". There is also a variant of this condition, seen approximately 10 to15% of the time. The hallmark of this variant is contralateral back pain following one or more ipsilateral back pain occurrences. This suggests that the various types of anatomy seen in the psoas muscle complex may respond differently to injury. The "rhomboid (upper back) recurrent back strain syndrome" is the most frequently syndrome seen in the upper back area. The majority of the time, this syndrome is associated with some type of "variable psoas pathology" of one leg. However, there is frequently not any lower back pain problems reported by the individual. The neck area generally involves the Trapezius Neck Strain Syndrome. Usually, psoas or rhomboid spasm is present, even though there are no reports of any significant "recurrent back strain syndromes" of the respective areas. If present, the key is to rehabilitate first the lower back and then the upper back. At this point, the neck muscles can be much more easily returned to a healthy condition.

Individuals with a "variable psoas pathology" also appear to have a high incidence of a hip click on this shortened side. A hip click is the snapping noise in the hip area when the leg is moved directly out to the side. I was 13 years old when I first noticed this popping noise in my right hip. Like many people in the 1960's, I was told this was a sign of hip damage and would probably lead to hip replacement at an early age unless I limited my activity. A sage father told me that he would "rather wear it out, rather than rust it out." This advice proved very valuable.

Fortunately in the 1980's, this problem of hip click was researched with ultrasound. It was shown conclusively to be a noise created by the snapping of the psoas minor or iliopsoas ligaments over the pelvic brim and had nothing to due with the hip joint. The pain in the hip appeared to be some type of referred pain. The final medical conclusion was that a hip click was a "completely benign process". However, the fact that the snap or click generally only exists on one side and not on the other, suggests something may not be quite right.

Opti-stretch research suggests that one possibility is a tightening of the psoas complex due to chronic spasm. The other possibility may be due to psoas tendon shortening. Individuals with hip clicks who repetitively engage in activities like martial arts, dance or rock climbing will frequently notice an increased soreness of that hip (due to radiated pain). Occasionally, groin pain will be reported. With proper Opti-stretch toning of the tight psoas complex, both the snap and discomfort from overuse can be significantly decreased. Unfortunately, seldom is this hip click noise completely eliminated.

If the chronically spasmed muscles can regain normal health, a large portion of the shortening can be reversed. However, if the tendon of the psoas complex (iliopsoas) has shortened, it appears that lengthening the tendon is at best extremely difficult and most likely not possible. Modern medicine teaches that other than surgery, tendon lengthening is virtually impossible. In this type of condition, it is imperative to maintain healthy muscle tone of the psoas complex muscles in order to prevent both injury and reinjury.

In summary, a large portion of the population has some type of measurable shortness of one leg (possibly up to 50 to 80%). Three separate causes of a short leg have been reported to exist (anatomical bone shortening, severe acute spasm of the psoas muscle and functional shortening). The anatomical short leg, where bone length is unequal, is quite common. Good clinical studies and Opti-stretch research both suggest there appears to be no significant increase in back pain associated with an anatomically shortened leg of less than approximately one inch. Whenever a leg is shorter, there is a lateral tilting of the pelvis. Without some type of compensation, the whole upper body would then tilt to one side. The spine responds by forming a rotational scoliosis or curvature of the spine, which can be either an S-shape or a C-shape.

If all the muscles of the back are healthy, the rotational scoliosis compensation occurs in the lumbar (lower) area of the spine. Due to the anatomy of the vertebrae in the lumbar region, rotational scoliosis can be very effectively compensated for and with minimal noticeable anatomic changes. However, if the psoas muscle complex of the lower spine is in some type of tightness or chronic spasm, the rotational scoliosis will then be compensated for primarily in the thoracic spine. The thoracic area of the spine area, due to the anatomy of the vertebrae, poorly compensates for rotational scoliosis. This frequently leads to a noticeable shoulder drop on one side or a significant kyphosis (hunchback). These two conditions are associated with the majority of the upper back and neck recurrent back strain syndromes that have been observed in the Opti-stretch research.

With regards to a "functional short leg," there exists at least some correlation from British studies that this particular condition may be associated with back pain problems. Opti-stretch research not only suggests that a chronic condition of leg shortening can exist due to chronic spasm and pathology of the psoas complex, but a true <u>syndrome</u> of various symptoms can be identified depending on the amount and severity of recurrent low back strains. Therefore, the term of a "psoas short leg syndrome" has been proposed and appears to be the major cause of recurrent low back strain. If there is documented functional shortening of less than 1/4 to 1/2 inch and if there are no recurrent back pain symptoms despite an active lifestyle, this condition is referred to as a "<u>psoas short leg trait</u>". This condition has been found in individuals with extremely healthy backs and often in the "never any back pain" group.

In my own experience, a 1-inch shortened right leg was diagnosed by an Orthopedic Surgeon at a premier Sports Medicine Clinic in the Northwest. I was given the choice of wearing a 1/2-inch insole (the largest lift that can be safely placed in a shoe) or the more recommended choice of building the sole of my right shoe up from the bottom by one inch. As I was having no problems at the time, I obviously chose the 1/2 inch custom insole lift and wore this type of lift religiously for 17 years. It was especially problematic for high performance ski boots, other high-tech athletic footwear and obeying the rule of having to take my shoes off, when I came into the house.

Following six months of Opti-stretch, the right leg length difference was only 3/16th of an inch and the lift was discontinued. The 1-inch difference did return on two separate occasions following significant injuries to the left hamstring. The shortening of the right leg was not readily noticeable. Due to the prolonged healing of the left hamstring injury, the shortening of the right leg was fortuitously detected. The right leg difference returned to 3/16th of an inch over a few weeks with Opti-stretch therapy. After happening a second time, it became apparent that the right leg shortening was extremely insidious, and appeared to influence the course of healing on the opposite limb. Opti-stretch research has shown that psoas injury, resultant spasm and consequential shortening of the one leg is a hallmark of the "psoas short leg syndrome" and the associated recurrent back strain episodes.

Also, this data supports that less than 1/4 to 1/2 inch difference in leg length can be compatible with a very healthy back if the muscles are optimally toned. After the above two experiences, a reliable method of simple documentation of any leg length difference was then developed. This method of leg measurement is called a Height-o-gram and is described in Appendix A.

The following sections of this book describe in detail, the incredible complexity of psoas muscle complex anatomy and physiology. Also, additional research and discovery are presented, supporting the association between the psoas muscle complex and recurrent back strain.

14. The Psoas Muscle

Anatomy

The psoas complex is a complex combination of three separate muscles. The psoas major muscle, the psoas minor muscle and the iliopsoas muscle. The psoas major and psoas minor muscles have their origin near the diaphragm in the chest cavity and travel along the antero-lateral vertebrae from T11 to L5 (from the diaphragm to the pelvis). Both then form fusiform muscles that travel over the iliacus muscle and is no longer attached closely to bone. From an anatomy standpoint this area of the muscle would be the weakest and most susceptible to injury. This area lies just deep to the sacroiliac joint area (to be discussed later). Both muscles travel over the iliacus muscle down the back wall of the pelvis. In the lower pelvis, the psoas minor muscle inserts on the pubic bone. This muscle does not leave the true pelvis. In contrast, the psoas major fuses with the iliacus muscle in the lower pelvis and becomes the iliopsoas muscle. While anatomical considered as one muscle, the muscle fibers of each muscle are often divided by a septate fascia.

As the iliopsoas muscle travels outside the abdomen through the inguinal canal, the muscle then splits into two separate muscle segments at the level of the groin. Each segment attaches by muscle fiber or tendon to a slightly different part of the medial top of the femur called the lesser trochanter. Careful dissection of the iliopsoas muscle shows a fibrous septate partition that keeps the muscle fibers of the psoas and iliacus muscles separate. The iliacus muscle fibers separate and attach to the lesser trochanter either as muscle fibers or as a tendon. The psoas major muscle usually always forms at least a 1/2 inch tendon, which wraps slightly around the lesser trochanter to attach. It attaches to the lesser trochanter at a slightly different plane than does the iliacus portion. This could explain why the muscle fibers of the psoas appear to have more stress placed on them in various leg positions.

Also, a never before reported anatomical variation was noted. In certain cadavers, a significantly longer length of the tendonous attachments were observed, if an iliacus tendon was present. These anatomical differences, which appear to be genetically determined, help to explain the observed tendon shortening of the psoas muscle complex. In theory, the longer tendon will have more chance of shortening with injury. It also helps explain why there are various patterns of psoas muscle primary injury and re-injury. More is explained in the following section dealing with physiology.

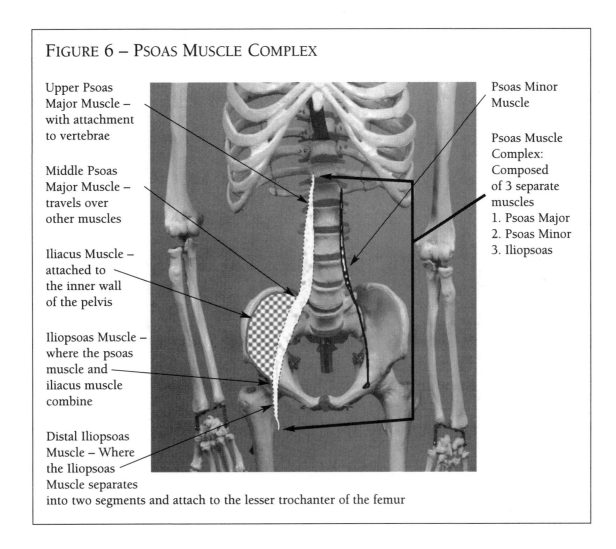

FIGURE 6 – PSOAS MUSCLE COMPLEX

Upper Psoas Major Muscle – with attachment to vertebrae

Middle Psoas Major Muscle – travels over other muscles

Iliacus Muscle – attached to the inner wall of the pelvis

Iliopsoas Muscle – where the psoas muscle and iliacus muscle combine

Distal Iliopsoas Muscle – Where the Iliopsoas Muscle separates into two segments and attach to the lesser trochanter of the femur

Psoas Minor Muscle

Psoas Muscle Complex: Composed of 3 separate muscles
1. Psoas Major
2. Psoas Minor
3. Iliopsoas

Anatomically this muscle and muscle complex are found in the majority of vertebrate life (except marine mammals). However, the exact anatomy and physiological function of the psoas complex muscles are completely unique in man, because man is the only species that walks fully erect.

The psoas minor muscle attaches to the lumbar vertebrae and travels down to attach to the pubic bone of the pelvis. It does not travel through the inguinal canal nor attach to the iliacus muscle. It has been documented by various authors to be absent in large percentages of various races (see Table 3, page 143). When absent, the psoas major muscle will sometimes send muscle fibers to attach to the pubic bone presumably to imitate the function of the psoas minor. The exact incidence of this anatomic occurrence has not been fully documented.

FIGURE 7 – ILIOPSOAS MUSCLE

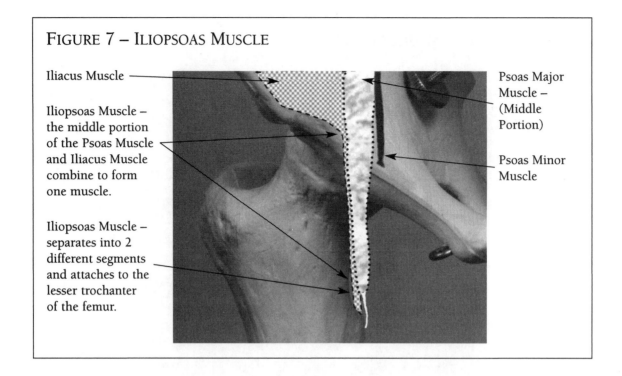

Iliacus Muscle

Iliopsoas Muscle –
the middle portion
of the Psoas Muscle
and Iliacus Muscle
combine to form
one muscle.

Iliopsoas Muscle –
separates into 2
different segments
and attaches to the
lesser trochanter
of the femur.

Psoas Major
Muscle –
(Middle
Portion)

Psoas Minor
Muscle

This describes only a small portion of the complexity of the muscles in the body appropriately referred to as the Psoas Complex. As you will see in the next section, the physiology of this muscle complex is even more "complex". This is in part because not everyone has the same configuration of these muscles.

PHYSIOLOGY

Anatomy books state that the psoas complex functions as both a weak lumbar stabilizer and a weak hip flexor. It also contributes in bending to the side. In beef, the psoas muscle complex is referred to as the tenderloin. It is present in all forms of terrestrial mammals. Because there are no other vertebrates besides man that walks erect, the precise function is difficult to investigate. Investigation in humans is nearly impossible due to its location along the anterior (front) part of the spine and covered by the contents of the abdominal cavity. As it dives deep in the pelvis, conventional means for the study of muscle function are not feasible.

Several papers trying to study the muscle have been written (Santaguida, P. L. and McGill, S. M. (1995) The psoas major muscle: A three-dimensional geometric study. J. Biomechanics). Each has concluded that this muscle is very difficult to study due to its location in the body. Also they report that the exact function is unknown.

To make matters even worse, there is tremendous anatomical variation in the presence or absence of the muscles, composing the psoas muscle complex. Studies show the psoas minor is absent either unilaterally or bilaterally in 56% of humans. This number varies according to race (personal communication with Dr. T.R. Olson).

TABLE 3 – PSOAS MINOR DATA

Psoas Minor Data – (references cited in the bibliography)

One study showed:
Psoas Minor
Present on both sides – 39 %
Present on the right – 7 %
Present on the left – 4 %
Absent on both sides – 50 %

Another study showed:
Complete Absence of the Psoas Minor Muscle
Russians – 48 %
Alsatians – 57 %
English – 59 %
Scotsmen – 63 %
Irish – 66 %
Blacks – 52.4 %
Chinese – 51.9 %

Another study showed:
The psoas minor muscle to be more frequently absent in males than females. John Bell (1793).

Another study showed:
The psoas minor muscle to be especially developed in leaping animals
such as the kangaroo, jerboa, macrocelides, etc.

This variation in the presence or absence of the psoas minor muscle is likely to be genetically linked. A commonly reported anatomical occurrence is when the psoas minor is absent, oftentimes a portion of the psoas major splits off and attaches to the pubic bone before entering the inguinal canal. The exact incidence has not been reported. Presumably, this variation is an attempt by the body to replace the missing psoas minor muscle.

Although more variations have been reported, there are at least three distinct anatomical forms the psoas muscle complex can exist in.

 A. **Psoas major only.**
 B. **Psoas major where a portion splits off and attaches to where the psoas minor would normally have attached.** (Note: this condition is reported but not significantly studied to determine the exact percentages.)
 C. **Psoas major and minor muscles present together (considered to be normal anatomy in humans).**

This means that some of the muscles of the Psoas Complex aren't even there half the time. For this reason, medical students are taught that the psoas complex has little function in back performance. There are other muscles in the body that are only present in half the population (i.e., pyramidalis, peroneus tertius, palmaris longus, and the plantaris). Each of the above mentioned muscles are much smaller muscles compared with the psoas complex. The classic muscle is the palmaris longus muscle of the forearm. In fact, I was taught in medical school that the only known function of the palmaris longus muscle was to provide tendon material so that plastic surgeons could operate. Opti-stretch theory suggests that the function of the psoas complex is grossly underestimated when it comes to back pain.

Opti-stretch research also suggests that the right side of the body is more commonly associated with <u>severe</u> recurrent back pain problems. The reason for this is unclear, but could possibly be associated with a dominant right hand or leg.

Assuming that the conditions A, B, and C above are roughly similar in proportion, and the side it occurs on is important, this would make nine possible anatomical combinations. If we then assume that the most stable back structures are those where the exact anatomy exists on both sides, there is only a 33% chance of not having back pain. Remember that these are only hypothetical assumptions.

Opti-stretch research has shown that there is a significant difference in the length when two tendons come off the distal psoas complex. It is assumed that the longer tendon on either the iliacus or psoas major may be more prone to tendon shortening and perpetuating a chronic injury state in the psoas complex. (Tendon shortening is, as previously stated, a significant clinical problem.) If you assume that only those individuals with completely identical anatomy on each side are less susceptible to injury, then approximately 17-33 % of the population would theoretically have low chance of having back pain. Factoring in serious back injury, these numbers are very close to the 20% of individuals in the United States population that never suffer from back pain. This suggests a population that, due to anatomy, is essentially "immune" from back pain unless affected by severe trauma or significant pathology. This group may also completely heal injured psoas major muscles without the formation of chronically injured muscles (ACIMs). These results also provide a hypothetical model as to why there are so many different forms of benign back pain (mild, moderate, and severe) and amount of injury, when the relative lifting or twisting stresses are often quite similar.

PAIN FROM THE PSOAS MUSCLE

Pain that originates from the psoas muscle also has a very unusual pattern. Direct pressure on the muscle or a relatively common infectious process on the surface of the muscle (called a psoas abscess) cause pain to be referred to the abdominal area. This is considered a normal referral pattern for this type of deep muscle. What has been overlooked in medicine is that, due to the tremendous complexity of the muscle, there might be other possible referral patterns.

In lower back pain, one of the more common locations of pain is over the sacroiliac joint (see Figure 1 – Posterior Back Anatomy, page 16). For over 30 years, both doctors and scientists have repeatedly looked at this location and at the sacroiliac joint. The majority of researchers conclude that pain over the sacroiliac joint is <u>not</u> due to injury or pathology of the sacroiliac joint itself. The overwhelming majority of data suggests that the sacroiliac joint is essentially immobile, except during pregnancy or unusual abnormalities. It is generally accepted that the sacroiliac joint does not play a role in common low back pain.

Millions of dollars have been spent researching this one specific area of low back pain because it is so common. Despite this extensive research, there has been no consensus as to **what actually does** cause this pain which has been recorded in this precise location for the past several hundred years.

The next anatomically deeper structures to the sacroiliac joint are the iliacus, psoas major and psoas minor muscles. The psoas muscles have not been thought to cause referred back pain for at least two reasons. First is the belief that the psoas muscles have little function when it comes to lifting motions performed by the back. Also, when an abscess forms in the front portion of the psoas muscle the pain is referred to the abdomen. This would suggest that the front half of the muscle radiates to the abdomen while the back part of the muscle radiates to the back. Given normal anatomy and physiology, this would be considered highly unlikely. However, structures deep in the chest and abdomen are not wired neurologically like the rest of the body. For instance a heart attack victim commonly describes pain in the jaw, shoulder or even the left little finger.

The best anatomical model for different types and locations of pain radiation is that of the abdominal aorta. This is the major blood vessel, which carries blood from the heart to the legs. Anatomically, it runs just in front of (anterior to) the psoas major muscle in the abdomen. They are both called retroperitoneal structures because they are deep to the peritoneal lining of abdominal cavity. In a disease state, the dissecting aortic aneurysm inner lining can separate from the outer lining. High-pressure blood can rush into this space and make the dissection worse. During the actual dissection, many patients complain of excruciating back pain (like someone is tearing their back out). Once the dissection has stopped, the patient then complains of severe <u>abdominal</u> pain. If the dissection again restarts, the excruciating pain resumes in the back. It is so painful that often the patient doesn't even complain of the abdominal pain. I had the opportunity of caring for several of these patients. I was always amazed with how excruciating the individual would describe the back pain and how rapidly it would subside once the acute dissection had stopped. Then complaints of abdominal pain would again resume.

Kidney infection and kidney stones are also classic examples of injury to structures in the retroperitoneal space and pain that is referred or radiated to the back. With kidney stones, the lower the location of the stone in the ureter, the lower the back pain.

Kidney stones very low in the ureter can cause abdominal pain on that same side once the ureter leaves the retroperitoneal space and enters the abdominal cavity.

In Anesthesiology Pain Management, several procedures require placing a needle safely through the back and into the retroperitoneal structures of the abdomen. Different approaches and paths are used to avoid the major nerves coming from the spine. The psoas muscle has the large femoral nerve running close to it. This and the location of other major nerves that exit from the spine make injection into this muscle extremely difficult. However, injecting the iliolumbar ligament of the back is a common technique in back pain rehabilitation. As mentioned above, the psoas complex lies directly deep to this structure. To insure that a needle could be passed through the iliolumbar ligament and safely into the psoas muscle, over 20 cadavers were dissected to insure no major nerves came close to this small area of the psoas. This research demonstrated the psoas muscle could be safely injected from the back. Injection of a lidocaine solution that will cause a minor burning sensation demonstrated that pain in the posterior or deep part of the psoas could cause referred pain to the back, at the injection site and the adjacent sacroiliac area as well.

A clinical technique for injecting the psoas, the iliopsoas, the iliacus and the hip extensors muscles was developed for evaluating the theories of Opti-stretch. These injections proved helpful in severely inflamed psoas complex states. This study suggests that the psoas muscle is the major contributor to back pain that is located over the sacroiliac joint area.

Another Opti-stretch study suggests the referred nature of this back pain. During severe back spasm due to myofascial strain, the pain is often in a band-like pattern and near the center of the spine. As the back heals over the next one to two weeks, the pain frequently changes to one side of the lower back area and often moves laterally to the area directly over the sacroiliac joint. After approximately a month, the constant pain even at rest is usually gone. However, upon bending backward at the low back level, even slightly, the sacroiliac pain will partially return. If a normal standing position is resumed, the pain goes away. This can be repeated multiple times. While in the standing erect position, there is no pain when pressing over the sacroiliac joint area. However, when the back is bent backwards and the pelvis tipped forward, the pain returns over the sacroiliac area. At this time, pressing over the sacroiliac area <u>does</u> cause an increase in pain. This pattern suggests that the pain sensation is actually coming from a referred source.

In summary, the differences in the psoas complex anatomy contribute to risk factors that play a key role in back pain. The psoas muscle itself can refer or radiate pain specifically over the sacroiliac joint area, one of the most common locations for lower back pain. Fortunately, Opti-stretch has shown that by first identifying and then correcting risk factors associated with the psoas complex, both the incidence and severity of recurrent low back pain decreases in those susceptible individuals.

FUNCTION WITH SPASM

Opti-stretch data suggests that the muscles of the psoas complex can partially spasm and shorten the leg at the hip joint. First with myself, the right leg was measured to be 1 inch shorter than the left leg. With 1 inch of leg length difference, it is easy to notice the disparity, once you know what to look for. Custom-made 1/2 inch insole lifts were worn in the right shoe for 17 years (which only partially accommodate this shortening). Following six months of Opti-stretch techniques, which led to marked improvement in range of motion, I noticed that the right leg felt different. Comparing the leg length, the right leg was about as long as the left. The insole lift was removed from the right shoe. Everything felt great for about 1 month. Preparing for a lecture and demonstration, I was lifting 200-pound barbells. A weight lifter informed me that weight lifters usually warm up with 250-pound barbells. As my back was feeling great, I rapidly worked up to 250 pounds. Upon lifting the weight for the second time, I felt a slight strain in my left hamstring. Over the coarse of the next six hours, the pain became severe.

It took almost one full month for the hamstring pain to reduce down to a mild level. I became quite disappointed that the injury was healing so slowly. I then fortuitously happened to note that the right leg was again approximately one inch shorter. I underwent steroid muscle injections and within a few days felt well enough to resume the Opti-stretch stretching exercises. Within two weeks, I felt great again and the right leg was very close to the same length as the left.

Several months later, while experimenting with stretch receptors, I accidentally sustained another severe left hamstring pull. This injury took several months to heal. Again the right leg was noted to be about one inch shorter than the left. Approximately two months after the injury, Opti-stretch prolotherapy injections were again received. Within a week, the leg felt well enough to resume the Opti-stretch routine. In a few weeks, the leg felt great and lifting heavy weights could again be resumed. This time the weight amount was very gradually and slowly increased to 200-pound barbells. After realizing the right leg could significantly shorten without being noticed, a new technique was devised to precisely measure the individual leg lengths. This technique is referred to as a height-o-gram (see Appendix A).

To use a height-o-gram, simply tape a piece of paper to the wall. A thick book (such as a phone book) is placed on the head and a pencil on top of the book. The hands are used to place the pencil lead and the book against the paper, which is taped to the wall. The individual's weight is slowly shifted from one leg to another. The easiest way is to lift the heel of the right foot leaving the toes barely touching in order to maintain balance. Then repeat the process on the opposite side. The difference between the height of the top and bottom of the curve was very consistent and gives an accurate measurement of any leg length difference.

Since that last injury, for a period of five years, the leg length difference has remained consistent at 3/16th of an inch. Only one significant moderate back strain has been sustained despite extremely aggressive lifting. Lifting a large 150 pound object from ground level, I experienced mild to moderate discomfort directly over both sacroiliac joints. No leg length shortening occurred.

FIGURE 8 – CORRECTED RIGHT SHOULDER DROP AND
PARTIAL CORRECTION OF THE RIGHT HIP DROP WITH OPTI-STRETCH.

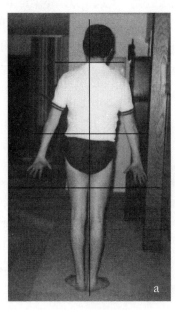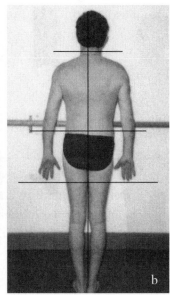

a. Back pose in 1997 prior to Opti-stretch and at the height of back problems. This pose was called the Statue of Liberty pose as all the muscles were contracted to stand as straight and tall as possible.

Note the significant drop of the right shoulder.

Also note the significant downward tilt of the right hip. This is due to a one inch shortening of the right leg.

b. Back pose in 1998. Back muscles were only partially contracted in this pose.

Note the marked correction of the right shoulder drop.

Also note there is still a visible angulation of the right hip downward due to a 3/16th inch shortening of the right leg. The right gluteus medius muscle has noticeably hypertrophied. Overall, there is fairly good symmetry of the upper back muscles.

CASE STUDIES EVALUATED WITH OPTI-STRETCH SCREENING EXERCISES

■ ■ ■

(Note: due to the acuteness of each injury these individuals were not treated with Opti-stretch.)

The next exciting body of data was generated with a near relative named Blake. Blake was the all-state offensive tackle for his High School championship team. At 6 ft. 2 inches, he also played varsity basketball. He was an excellent all around athlete. During his senior year, I had measured his leg length to measure angular movement of the ankle in an athlete. His leg length measurement showed a 1/4 inch shortening of the left leg with otherwise excellent body symmetry and range of motion.

FIGURE 9 – BLAKE 1 WEEK AFTER INJURY.

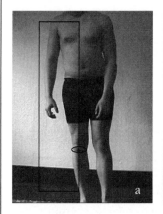 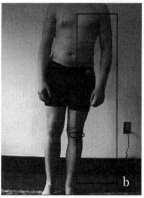

He was still uncomfortable when walking. The significant difference in movement when transferring weight from one leg to the other could easily be seen on videotape.

a. Upon weight transfer to the right leg, the upper body is shifted further over the leg. There is an angulation and slight rotation of the left side of the pelvis toward the front (anterior). Although not easily apparent, there is approximately a 3/4 inch lowering of the right pelvis suggesting a functional shortening of the right leg.
b. While standing on the left foot, there is less shift of the weight at the knee over the foot. There is also less shift to the left of the upper body.

Note the symmetrical circles at the knees. When the weight is transferred to the right leg, the body automatically compensates for the 3/4 inch shortening of the right leg. The body is able to compensate without the person even being aware of the difference.

Two months later he sustained a severe snowboard accident, where he fell striking his lower back area. The pain was severe and located over the right lower sacroiliac joint.

Back x-rays were normal at the Emergency Room and he was diagnosed with a muscle strain. On returning home, the left leg was measured. Instead of being 1/4 inch shorter than the right leg, it was now 3/4 inch longer than the right leg. Also, there was marked tenderness of the psoas, iliacus and iliopsoas muscles. Leg length measurements were performed every other day. The leg length difference stayed the same during six separate measurements. After two weeks, the pain started to subside to the point where Blake could walk standing straight up and without a limp. His leg length in a two-day period had changed from right leg being shorter by 3/4 inches to his pre-injury condition where the left leg was 1/4 inch shorter. This suggests during pain and spasm of the psoas muscle complex, one leg can become shortened by as much as one inch.

FIGURE 10 – BLAKE'S HIP ROTATION.   1 WEEK AFTER SNOWBOARD INJURY.

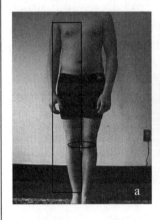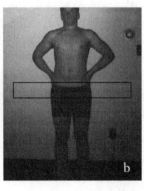

a. There is a significant amount of left shoulder anterior rotation. (Notice how the left hand has moved in front of the left leg.) The right hip appears slightly shorter at the belt line. Note that the shoulder height is roughly the same given the anterior rotation of the left shoulder.
b. The tips of the thumbs are placed on the anterior superior iliac spines. A significant lowering of the right hip area can be seen.

Note: Precise measurements are difficult from photography alone due to the complex combinations of movement in the human body. The photograph converts a 3 dimensional image into a 2 dimensional image making subtle anterior rotations appear slightly larger.

Conservative walking activity was all Blake was comfortable with due to the pain. Due to the acute injury, Opti-stretch exercises were not recommended. By six weeks, he gradually reported feeling back to normal. However, he was still unable to get comfortably down into a squatting position (something easily performed prior to the injury). At eight weeks, the squatting position had returned to normal, yet he still had mild back discomfort on trying to perform a bridge. Over the next couple of weeks he resumed playing both football and tennis. A month later, the bridge was completed without back discomfort.

In the young healthy 18-year-old athlete, the problem partially corrected itself with the healing of the back injury. Unknown to either one of us was the significant drop in

FIGURE 11 – BLAKE 8 MONTHS AFTER BACK INJURY.

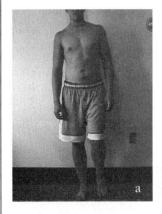 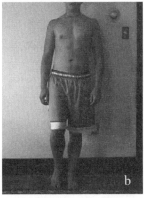

a. Standing on the right leg. Note the significant upper body shift to the right. There is a marked lowering of the right shoulder

b. Standing on the left leg. The upper body is more aligned compared to the other photo. Note there is still a slight lowering of the right shoulder. Ideally the right shoulder should be slightly raised. The arms hang much more symmetrically compared to one week after the injury.

FIGURE 12 – BLAKE'S SHOULDER DROP. 8 MONTHS AFTER SNOWBOARD INJURY.

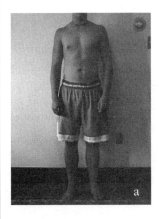 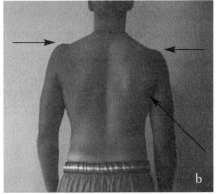

a. Standing on both legs. Note the significant drop of the right shoulder.
b. Posterior view of the right shoulder drop and the difference in how the scapula appears.

the right shoulder height. This suggests that although the back had apparently healed, there is a high probability that some of the back muscles had not completely healed and had stayed in a chronic injury state. Shoulder height asymmetry such as this has frequently been observed for individuals suffering from "recurrent back pain syndromes", especially associated with psoas injury.

Two other examples were noted to support the concept of spasm of the psoas muscle and the diagnostic value of Opti-stretch. Both were females of about 17 years of age.

They were cousins. They were both extremely athletic and both could easily complete all of the advanced Opti-stretch stretching exercises without difficulty and with full range of motion. Each would be considered very flexible. Dayna had a 1/4 inch shorting of her left leg. The right leg of Sasha also measured 1/4 inch shorter. Within a two-year period of time both of them had sustained a moderate back strain. Each had approximately 1/4 inch further shortening of the respective legs at the time of the moderate back pain. Opti-stretch screening stretches showed a full two inch inability to complete the "Sitting Nose to Knee" – (Figure Four) on their respective shortened sides. Several other significant differences in body symmetry were found using the screening stretches. After resolution of the moderate back pain, the screening stretches were then repeated. The symmetrical range of motion had completely returned. Also, the leg length on the respective sides returned to 1/4 inch difference.

Data from these three individuals suggests that, at least in certain individuals, shortening of one leg can occur with injury. This was associated with low back pain and psoas muscle complex tenderness. With healing of the back injury, the shortening returned to pre-injury length.

15. UPPER BACK PAIN AND THE RHOMBOID MUSCLES

This topic was covered previously. Briefly, the rhomboid area is the area most commonly associated with recurrent upper back pain. If someone deeply massages between the shoulder blades, the difference in tenderness can often be felt. By performing the rhomboid pull about as strong as one can, this will produce muscle tenderness on the chronically injured side. The rhomboid muscles are difficult to stretch due to the shoulder girdle. Therefore, the muscles may be toned by isotonic and isometric contraction. Tightening these muscles and pulling the shoulder blades together is one of the most consistent types of involuntary stretches seen in man.

16. NECK PAIN AND THE TRAPEZIUS MUSCLES

The neck stretching exercises presented in Opti-stretch are quite basic but very effective in detecting asymmetry. Only after first correcting the lower back, upper back and shoulder asymmetry, can these rather common and simple stretches be sufficient to correct most problems of the trapezius muscle. Spasm of the trapezius muscle was found to be commonly associated with recurrent neck pain on the same side. Unfortunately, the neck is very complex and easily injured. **Never exceed the mild discomfort intensity level**. If the Opti-stretch program does not significantly improve the recurrent neck strain problem, return to the physician who performed your pre-Opti-stretch physical, for re-evaluation.

17. SHOULDER HEIGHT AND ASYMMETRY

Uneven shoulder height is very common in the general population and generally goes completely unnoticed. This condition can easily be detected by simply looking in the mirror and marking the top of each shoulder with a grease pencil. Then take a level and draw horizontal lines through each point. The difference in height can be measured with a ruler. More than a 1/2 inch difference often means that something might be wrong with the hips, lower back or upper back.

An extremely accurate measurement of shoulder rotation is the "Finger Touch" stretching exercise. With one hand placed behind the back and the other placed behind the head attempt to touch the fingers. If there is more than a 1-inch difference from left to right, then measure how high up the back each hand will reach. Next measure how far down the back each hand will reach to determine where the tightness is in the shoulders. Frequently, I will hear the comment that "everybody has a difference". This can easily be demonstrated not to be true in at least 20% of the population. However, there can be a 1-inch difference with excess activities using a dominant arm.

The next common statement is; "Oh yeah, I broke that clavicle (or separated that shoulder) years ago". Utilizing the Opti-stretch program, several of these individuals have not only been able to decrease the asymmetry in range of motion but also regain function that had been lost for decades. If there is any asymmetry of more than 1 inch, seriously consider the Opti-stretch program shoulder stretches. If you can't come within 1 inch on the "Finger touch", also seriously consider giving Opti-stretch a try. You might be pleasantly surprised. An A-C separation shoulder injury from long ago may return to essentially normal. To be able to skip a rock or throw a baseball again without pain is great.

18. CHIROPRACTIC AND OTHER MANIPULATIONS

Manipulation is simply defined as any operation "done by hand". In carefully observing the majority of manipulation techniques, such as Osteopathy and Physical Therapy, what essentially is being done is that the therapist is stretching your muscles for you. This is often referred to as direct manipulation.

Indirect manipulation is generally practiced by chiropractors. Often one joint or muscle is stretched in order to provide relief to another injured muscle or nerve.

Spinal manipulation dates back to the time of Hippocrates. Various manuscripts from early Egyptian, Greek, Chinese and Hindu reveal that certain types of chiropractic treatment have been around since the early beginnings of man. Bone manipulation was practiced in the Middle Ages. A type of chiropractic technique was noted in the Native American Indians, when they had the children walk barefoot on a painful back to help relieve the pain.

"The Father of Chiropractic" is recognized as Dr. D. D. Palmer, who in 1895 performed the first documented chiropractic manipulation in the USA. Described in the literature as a "frontier renaissance man", he was a schoolteacher, farmer and Iowa grocer who first started practicing under the title of a "Magnetic Healer". In the early years of Chiropractic, the "lumbar roll" was developed. The precise physiologic process behind the technique has eluded investigators both in and out of the Chiropractic profession.

This single technique called the "lumbar roll" has evolved as a mainstay for the profession. In the 1980's, there was a significant fervor for trying to solve the mystery of the lumbar roll's "million dollar pop". A million dollars was offered to anyone who could explain the "pop" and why it was effective. Since the 1980's, the physiological theory behind "the pop" has generally become accepted as a process of "cavitation". This means that pressure on the joint can displace small amounts of dissolved nitrogen gas causing a "pop". The gas is then reabsorbed over the following hour. This appears to be a normal physiological function of the joints to displace acute stress forces.

There are a number of things that are known about the "lumbar roll":

1. Early high velocity techniques suggest that the manipulation does not directly involve the severely spasmed and injured psoas muscles of common severe low back strain. However, by relaxing major hip flexor muscles (accessory muscles of the psoas complex), the "lumbar roll" indirectly helps to reduce the spasm and pain in the psoas muscles.
2. It first evolved as a high velocity, high-energy manipulation of the lumbar spine. Today, low velocity and moderate velocity manipulation are used with equal efficacy.
3. Chiropractors formally teach that the manipulation is the essential ingredient and not the "pop". Therefore, an equally efficient manipulation is obtained with and without the "pop". Manipulation of a healthy spine demonstrates that a "pop" is often difficult to generate.

I have watched many skilled Chiropractic physicians perform the "lumbar roll". I also spent approximately 200 hours in one of the finest libraries of anatomy that I have ever seen, which was incidentally at a College of Chiropractic. I also enrolled as a "guinea pig" at the College of Chiropractic to have student's practice on me. Having also studied aspects of manipulation from various other medical sciences, I have proposed a plausible theory.

Opti-stretch theory suggests that:

1. The "pop" appears indeed to be consistent with a theory like cavitation. A simple demonstration of cavitation is the following. If one fully flexes the fingers toward the wrist (without any assistance), the distance can easily be noted with a pen mark. Then, if an average individual "pops" their knuckles, the fingers will be able to flex 2 millimeters further. Over the next hour, the fingers will

not "pop" again. After at least a one-hour rest, the fingers can no longer flex to the longer distance. However, upon "popping" the fingers again, the two millimeters further range of motion is restored.

This suggests that the cushion of dissolved nitrogen gases provides a safety valve so that when a stress occurs, the release of this safety valve allows for increased range of motion and less trauma to the joint and its musculo-skeletal structures. This provides further joint movement, allowing the spasmed muscles of the spine to partially relax and therefore helps relieve pain (usually at least an hour). Even partial relaxation of the muscle may help to break the "pain – spasm cycle" of back pain and provide the patient with some pain relief.

2. The muscle groups primarily stretched during the "lumbar roll" are the major hip flexor muscles of which there are at least six. The fact that there are many muscles serving the same function makes it less likely to injure any one specific muscle. As described previously, when a muscle is strained or sprained, it tends to go into spasm. If the injury is severe enough, accessory muscles will help out by going into spasm to further immobilize the joint. If the injury is extremely severe, the antagonistic muscles will then also spasm to provide maximum immobilization of the bone or joint.

The antagonist muscles in the Opti-stretch theory are the erector spinae muscles of the spine. In severe back strain, they are tender to the touch and have marked knots and spasm. I learned that as a physical therapy aide, over a week or two, through diathermy and massage, the erector spinae muscles could easily be relaxed. These erector spinae muscles would clinically appear to be back to normal healthy muscle tissue to the touch (knots, tenderness, and tightness were gone). However, only the severe back pain would be improved. The mild and moderate back pain would still require additional weeks of therapy to heal the back completely.

The back pain would be expected to persist because the psoas complex muscles were severely injured and have not yet completely healed (which usually takes one to two months no matter what therapy is employed). The accessory muscles of the psoas complex are the major hip flexor muscles. These muscles are in <u>reflex spasm</u> but not individually injured. By taking the major hip flexor muscles through the given range of motion of the "lumbar roll" the spasm of these muscles is partially broken. Partial spasm relief and subsequent pain relief of accessory muscles will trigger some relaxation of the antagonist muscles of the lumbar spine. If this is done every day or every other day, the severe pain is reported by many individuals to disappear faster than without therapy.

3. This explains why individuals are prompted (by the return of pain and by their Chiropractic physician) to return on a frequent basis following acute injury.

4. This may help to explain why 19.5 million people in the United States annually go to chiropractors. They feel they get faster relief of their severe pain symptoms. Anything that helps take away the <u>severe pain</u> of back spasm, even for 24 hours is a welcome relief. Once all the <u>severe</u> pain is gone, the average person doesn't focus quite so much on the length of time it takes to completely heal the injury.

5. This also explains why traditional medicine has analyzed the results over and over in very sophisticated studies and has found there is no faster healing of a severely injured back when Chiropractic is employed.

19. Dyspareunia

Dyspareunia is one-sided abdominal pain in females during intercourse. It appears to be a mechanical stimulation of pain fibers, particularly when significantly extra stress is placed off the midline plane or if other rather significant forces are generated. Generally, this condition is alleviated by a complete gynecological work-up. However, several individuals were referred to our Pain Management Clinic, as the source of the pain could not be found. I was impressed at the similarity of each story and how devastating it was for them and their families. All had undergone extensive tests and even exploratory abdominal surgery to leave no stone unturned in this serious problem.

At that time, the Pain Management Clinic had nothing to offer these unfortunate women. Now, at least in theory, Opti-stretch may be helpful. With Opti-stretch, we know the psoas complex can be very tender if these muscles are palpated while in a chronic injury state. Due to the depth of the psoas muscle in the pelvis, the presumably affected segment of psoas cannot be palpated. However, both above and below this area the psoas complex can usually be easily palpated for tenderness, especially in females with near ideal body weight.

Anatomically, both the ovary and the uterus are partially attached directly over the psoas muscle. Therefore, significant movement of these female organs could cause abdominal discomfort from the anterior surface of the psoas muscle if the individual had an asymptomatic chronically injured psoas muscle (ACIM). By using Opti-stretch toning of the psoas muscle complex, the muscle becomes less tender to palpation. Whether this might help in certain cases where every other form of therapy has failed is unknown. However, for those brave enough to undergo surgery to evaluate the problem, a couple of months of stretching exercises, if indicated, may well be worth the effort in "leaving no stone unturned".

20. ARTHRITIS

There are some reports by participants in Opti-stretch that minor common arthritic problems are either improved or eliminated. These individuals also noted a decrease in the sensation of stress in the joints.

Movement and anti-inflammatory medications are the most commonly recommended forms of therapy for all common (degenerative) arthritis. Opti-stretch theory proposes that, by lengthening the stretch receptors and rehabilitating tight muscles, the joint moves with less stress. This lessening of the stress allows healing of the inflamed joint tissue, which is a definite part of arthritis. Whether Opti-stretch may be of some help in moderate or severe arthritic conditions is doubtful and has not yet been evaluated.

Also, of note, is the observation that moderate and severe arthritic conditions have shown to be a significant impediment to re-toning injured muscles (ACIMs).

21. POSTURE

Besides improving recurrent back pain problems, the most exciting results from Opti-stretch have been the improvement in posture. Posture is again a very complex subject and can have many causes for any given abnormality. Many people usually do not pay much attention to posture unless the individual they see has either very good posture or very poor posture. Frequently an individual is unaware that they are beginning to develop noticeably poor posture.

A common type of poor posture is the rounding of the shoulders forward. This is generally due to a kyphosis or forward rounding of the upper back. The head is then generally carried in a forward tilt position. There are several causes of this problem. One is a true scoliosis of the spine. Another is due to a "rotational" scoliosis of the spine. A common cause of a rotational scoliosis is functional shortening of one leg. While insole lifts tend to help the problem somewhat, the condition frequently progresses to the point that in old age, it can be a serious problem. Gravity and the normal aging process both make the problem more severe.

Another very common problem with posture is the drop of one shoulder. Determination of this problem was previously described. If looked for, it can usually be both easily seen and precisely measured.

An interesting occurrence is that frequently individuals with even 1 full inch of "bone shortening" of the leg do not exhibit rounding of the shoulders or a drop in height of one shoulder. In fact, athletic individuals with 1 inch of bone shortening often have extremely good posture.

Opti-stretch theory suggests that leg shortening due to psoas tightening ("variable psoas pathology") causes different forces to be exerted on the spine. In individuals with an anatomical short leg, the major part of the rotation of the spine occurs in the lower back area, which is structured to compensate for this rotational stress. However, with functional shortening and the associated psoas tightness and tenderness, the lower back does not rotate as much. The psoas extends all the way up to T11 which is in the mid back area. This lack of rotation in the lower back therefore places the rotational forces on the upper spine and stress on the shoulders. The upper back and neck vertebrae do not accommodate well to these rotational forces. Therefore, these forces cause an increased rounding of the upper spine and dropping of one shoulder. This condition can contribute to upper back and neck recurrent strains.

If permanent changes have not occurred, the posture is often remarkably improved following completion of the Opti-stretch program. The rounding of the upper back and shoulders can actually return to a near normal appearance even after 25 years of having rounded shoulders. The head tilt is also significantly lessened. One thing is certain. If you have poor posture and it hasn't been improved or corrected by Opti-stretch, a medical evaluation is probably recommended.

If you ever have been told to stand up straight by your mother, or by a friend that thinks you may be slouching a little, consider lateral photographs and shoulder height determinations to demonstrate your normal posture. If there is a problem, see if you can improve it with Opti-stretch.

22. "Dr. Mom"

The largest numbers of primary care providers in the world are affectionately referred to as "Dr. Mom". They are the first to evaluate the sprained ankles and strained backs. They either treat or refer to the medical doctor. The advice for mild back strains from the average mother "Dr. Mom" has always been to give a back strain a little rest and avoid lifting any heavy objects. After a period of time to heal the injury, they advise gradually working oneself back to normal activity and to be more careful the next time. Modern medicine has come full circle. In the 1960's and early 70's, most patients with severe common back pain were hospitalized and placed in bed rest with continuous traction. This proved neither medically beneficial nor cost effective. Today, medical therapy significantly concurs with the age-old advice of "Dr. Mom". Extensive medical data shows that the majority of common back pain cases will get better in one to two months regardless of whether physical therapy, chiropractic medicine or no treatment at all is employed. It appears that nothing will consistently hasten the normal healing process of a severe back strain.

Until Opti-stretch, there hasn't been a good precise plan for gradually working oneself back to 100% activity or even knowing when full activity should be tried. With Opti-stretch, you will know your range of motion before the injury. Once this same range of motion is comfortably achieved, the muscles are ready to strengthen and condition. Upon completing these three steps, 100% activity is usually safe. More importantly, if a child or young adult cannot comfortably reach their before-injury range of motion, then 100% effort in activity level is not advisable.

Opti-stretch has also been designed particularly for "Dr. Mom", with regards to posture problems. In the past, their only advice for posture problems was to <u>repetitively</u> tell their child to "**stand up straight**". Now there exists a better way. With the Opti-stretch screening program, they can actually demonstrate if there are any asymmetries in the muscular function of their child's back. By encouraging the relatively simple Intermediate Therapeutic Program, many of the postural problems can be improved. If certain goals are achieved and the problem still exists, a formal medical consultation may be indicated.

One of the most exciting prospects is the routine testing on a periodic basis using the Advanced Program. By starting at "3 to 5" years of age, Dr. Moms might be able to help ensure that their child can obtain a good solid range of motion for virtually any activity that the child desires throughout adolescence. Those individuals that have preserved this range of motion into adulthood and even older age, are generally more active and have better health.

In the past, many children would try extremely hard "to excel" in sports. However, due to the fact that they had tight muscles or chronically injured muscles, they had to work twice as hard as the other kids. Also, they were the ones most likely to sustain injuries. This unfortunately can lead to decreased interest in an active lifestyle as the adolescent matures.

The most exciting goal is the potential for decreasing the epidemic of back pain. Every "Dr. Mom" knows directly or indirectly someone who suffers from some type of back pain. In the United States, it is a serious and incapacitating epidemic. Opti-stretch does not protect against every type of back pain. However, statistically, these other types of pathologic back pain account for less than 15% of the individuals who suffer from back pain.

Opti-stretch is designed only for common back pain due to strained muscles. However, the statistical probability that an adolescent or young adult will experience some type of noticeable muscular back strain is extremely high. Those who are able to establish and then preserve optimal muscle tone to the core muscles of the spine, two things generally occur. First, the severity of muscle strains tends to decrease. Second, the chances of various recurrent back pain syndromes are significantly decreased. A <u>major goal</u> of Opti-stretch is to decrease "recurrent back pain syndromes" in our children's lifetime.

Asymmetric muscle tightness is a risk factor and significantly increases the chance of injury to muscles of the spine. In my experience as a practicing physician and doing sports physicals, only 10 to 20% of primary school children had potentially correctable muscle tightness of some type. About 20-40% of middle school teenagers had this type of problem. By high school over 50-70% of the students had asymmetric muscle tightness. Note that these individuals examined were primarily the "athletes" of the school. The younger the child, the more rapidly tight muscles can be corrected. The optimum time is while the bones are still growing and shaping (usually before age 18).

Protection and prevention are very realistic goals for "Dr. Mom" to implement using the Opti-stretch program. (Also a word of advice, it's always better for Dr. Mom to demonstrate to the child the exercises rather than to simply just teach them.) Other goals and benefits include:

1. Protect against back injury.
2. Protect against reinjury to an already injured muscle while it is healing.
3. To be able to determine when an injured muscle is healed and ready for full activity.
4. Prepare adolescents for the "weekend warrior syndrome".
5. Tone muscles.
6. Shape muscles.
7. Improve posture.
8. Screen for problems in children who are not performing in sports as well as expected, given the amount of effort and practice.
9. Retain a child-like mobility for life.

23. CONCLUSION

The month of October is set aside as "Family Health Month". "Stay Active!" "Stay fit!" The epidemic of back pain is a major cause of decreased activity levels in all parts of the world today. Many unfortunate sufferers of recurrent back pain find that after the second or third reoccurrence, they either consciously or subconsciously scale back on their level of activity. For many, this is quite effective. Many who scale back to only the activities of daily living find a significant decrease in recurrent back pain unless this level of activity is exceeded.

While a decreased level of activity is acceptable for some, the majority of individuals have a strong desire for a more active lifestyle. These individuals are sensible in trying to maximize the protection of their back. Often, they can even gradually work up to some very impressive activity levels. However, once every one to five years the right combination of stresses occurs to cause a recurrent back strain.

Until Opti-stretch, only a relatively small percentage of individuals with recurrent back strain syndrome have found the right combination of exercises to regain a completely healthy back. The major reason is that the core muscles of the back are extremely difficult to strengthen and condition unless there is at least a certain level of toning of the muscles. Trying to strengthen tight and chronically injured muscles without first toning the muscles, frequently leads to reinjury.

Presented in this book are the major types and locations of recurrent back pain that are due solely to muscle strain. Realize that if your history of back pain is not similar to the described examples, you may have something other than benign back pain. More importantly, just because you have what appear to be ACIMs does not rule out other more serious underlying pathology. Anyone who has had even a single episode of moderate or severe back strain should consult a medical doctor.

Opti-stretch specifically identifies tight and chronically injured muscles due to muscle strain. The stretching exercises are scientifically designed to tone the core muscles of the back, which are most commonly responsible for recurrent low back pain. The "gold standard" and major goal of Opti-stretch, is to return your muscles to the same tone you enjoyed as a "3 to 5 year old".

Why is the average range of motion of a "3 to 5 year old" set as the "gold standard"? After all, many professional athletes and individuals with very healthy backs cannot reach the "gold standard". Remember that range of motion is largely hereditary and related to body type. However, once a recurrent strain syndrome has occurred, it may be necessary reach the "gold standard" to completely re-tone the chronically injured muscles. Currently, there is no evidence suggesting that <u>further</u> range of motion beyond the level of a normal "3 to 5 year old" is significantly beneficial for a healthy back in most normal individuals. (Recall, this may not prove to be the case in the hyperflexible group.)

It is well known that if there is no range of motion of the muscles or joints, there is no "activity" level. Even small increases in range of motion toward normal can have profound increases in activity level. Next, we know that there are large groups of individuals with excessive range of motion. This group often suffers from high incidence of recurrent back and hip pain. Somewhere between these two extremes there appears to be an optimum range of motion or "gold standard". Flexibility steadily decreases from birth. Between ages "3 to 5", 95% of healthy children can easily perform all of the exercises in the Advanced Stretching Program. By age 5, flexibility takes one of three different pathways. Either flexibility continues to decrease (common in most males), flexibility can stay the same, or flexibility can increase (common in many females).

Of the 2000 individuals interviewed, approximately 400 (most over the age of 40) were in the "never had any back pain" category. Many had some mild asymmetry but the majority were quite symmetrical. Their range of motion either equaled or was within 3 or 4 inches of the "gold standard" for every exercise in the Advanced Program (with the exception of the "Bridge"). However, those individuals with recurrent low back strain syndromes could not complete the Advanced Program stretching exercises and frequently demonstrated significant asymmetry of between 1 to 8 inches.

The next breakthrough in Opti-stretch came with taking a previously very inflexible athletic male and restoring him through six months of Opti-stretch to the "gold standard" level. Fortunately, the back pain decreased in proportion. Remember, if a 45-year-old who experienced tight muscles since adolescence can reach the "gold standard"; **you probably can too**! This is an extremely exciting discovery of the Opti-stretch program.

If you were a normal "3 to 5 year old", you were at the "gold standard" level. Therefore, with the proper amount of work and over sufficient time, Opti-stretch has shown that the "gold standard" is indeed a realizable goal. Even if you are unable to reach this level, every inch of stretch receptor lengthening accomplished allows the core muscles of the back to become more toned, more symmetrical and therefore more healthy.

Chronically painful joints and other types of chronically painful tissue send signals to the muscles to change into their protective or spasm mode. While gentle Opti-stretch may be helpful, this is one condition that has proven to be extremely problematic.

Opti-stretch is an exciting new stretching exercise program for ages 6 to 86. If you perform the Screening Program and can find no risk factors, and if you consider yourself to be a healthy athletic type of individual, give the Advanced Program for Fit Athletes and Children a try. If you can perform these stretching exercises, you are either in or very close to the 20% of the population who are at little or no significant risk for recurrent back strain.

Now that you have read the book, you owe it to yourself to at least give the Screening Program a try. Located in Appendix C is a sample of results from my Intermediate Screening Test and measurements after my Intermediate Therapeutic Program. Completion of the screening tests is the first step of the **Opti-stretch Challenge**. On a comfortable exercise mat or thick carpet, sit down and record **your own results**. Remember that you only stretch to your own comfort level. The intensity of stretch must be the same for both sides and it has to be held for at least 5 seconds (30 seconds is even better). All the stretches do not have to be completed at one session. When you finish, if you do not have any risk factors in the Beginning or Intermediate Tests consider the Advance Program for Fit Athletes and Children. If you can pass this program chances are extremely high that you have well toned core muscles in your back and you have passed the final step of the Opti-stretch Challenge. Keep the results, these measurements can prove extremely useful in the rehabilitation of an unfortunate severe injury like a fall or auto accident. Also, the stretching exercises can be repeated between every six months to every five years to assure nothing has changed and that the core muscles of the back are aging gracefully. Also, these stretching exercises should be performed after healing any significant injury to either the extremities or the back. This will detect whether there might have been some incomplete healing in the core muscles of the spine, which can easily go unnoticed.

If you do happen to detect any risk factors, consider eliminating them with a two to six month Opti-stretch Intermediate Therapeutic Program, which is the second step in the Opti-stretch Challenge. (If any of the stretches seemed difficult just getting into the starting position go directly to the Beginning Program for at least two months.) Then, give the Advanced Program a try. The third and final step of the Opti-stretch Challenge, is the Maintenance Program. You will then know that you have successfully turned over one more stone in your battle against recurrent back pain.

Good luck with Opti-stretch! I sincerely hope it will be as beneficial to you as it has been to others.

Please try to be fair when assessing the Opti-stretch technique. If you haven't read portions of the book at least twice, feel comfortable with the information and possibly haven't attended a seminar or received one-on-one instruction, then you may not be doing Opti-stretch correctly.

Opti-stretch is designed to be a very precise program. This allows trouble-shooting if there are problems and identification of individuals who might indeed be dealing with a pathologic problem rather than simply a muscle strain problem. First, it is imperative you record your range of motion measurements. The initial and one to two month re-measurements are essential. Second, choose a daily routine. The minimum is two stretches (Figure Four) and (Butterfly). Third, mark on the calendar when you stretch. As mentioned earlier, if there are significant lapses, you should restart your two-month program interval. It is difficult to emphasize enough these three simple steps if you are going to try the program and realistically expect the results that are possible with Opti-stretch.

Opti-stretch was designed for relatively healthy individuals with no significant medical problems. However, if you have made an honest attempt at learning all of the concepts and principles in Opti-stretch and as a healthy individual, you have still sustained an injury, this is something that needs to shared with others and myself. There is a good possibility that there are groups of individuals who, for whatever reason, may not tolerate Opti-stretch. Examples might be those individuals with extremely low or high pain thresholds. Also, there may be groups of individuals that for some reason are not able to properly feel a residual stretching sensation after the stretch has been completed. This could possibly be due to a mild neuropathy. These individuals may have to change to some other program.

If you happen to have an adventuresome spirit, make sure that if you make any modifications of the Opti-stretch technique or the Opti-stretch stretching exercises, please refer to it as your own technique. As an example, take (Figure Four) for instance. This exact stretching exercise can be performed standing, sitting, supine and inverted. Only two of the four ways are safe for the Opti-stretch technique.

A great deal of time and effort has gone into trying to make Opti-stretch both an effective and safe program. In the early days of Opti-stretch, I was extremely enthusiastic about the potential of the program. Approximately, 20 different physicians were approached about their opinions. This ranged from general practitioners, to major University professors, and even to a medical society. The majority had no real interest when they were told it dealt with stretching exercises as the basis for correcting back pain. In all fairness to these physicians, it is difficult to condense all of the information contained in this book into a 20-minute conversation or a letter. Also, a few new theories have only recently evolved to explain various results following years of testing.

I will always remain impressed by one fellow physician's comments. He patiently listened to about a 45-minute presentation. Then he simply stated, "Even if your theories are right, you can't make any money at this as a physician". He was 100% correct. There is no way an average physician can instruct an individual in the Opti-stretch techniques due to the time constraints. However, two or three of the stretching exercises would make excellent screening techniques for certain types of physicians and health care providers. This is in part why the program had to at least be tested for several years.

There are reasons why stretching exercises have continued to exist for thousands of years. There are also reasons why traditional medicine has not completely accepted any one technique with the exception of Physical Therapy. Hopefully, after reading the book you will have a different insight as to why controversies exist.

Not only has time been invested, but also a great deal of personal sacrifice has occurred directly as a result of my enthusiasm to study this information and share it with others. Mild and moderate recurrent back pain syndromes often do not cause major lifestyle changes. However, "severe recurrent back pain syndrome" can be very devastating both mentally and physically. Moreover, statistically there may exceed over one million individuals suffering with this severe condition in the USA alone. If Opti-stretch can prevent the decades of needless back pain and incapacity that I experienced, in even a handful of individuals, then the sacrifices will have been worth it.

> Very Best of Luck in Achieving Your Own Personal
> Goals for a healthy back and an active lifestyle.

OVERVIEW

■ ■ ■

1. Back pain has now reached epidemic proportions and needlessly millions of lives are negatively effected.

2. If you are above age 30 and have <u>never</u> experienced back pain you are likely in the 20% of the population that probably will not have any back pain in their entire lifetime. (A tremendous <u>genetic benefit</u>)

3. However, if you have experienced two or more episodes of a strained back in precisely the same place, you have by definition "<u>recurrent back pain</u>". Even one episode of <u>severe low back pain</u> can place you in a high-risk category for "recurrent back pain".

4. If you have several <u>risk factors</u>, the likelihood of recurrences of back pain is extremely high, depending on the activity level of the lifestyle that you choose.

5. Now there is a <u>screening test</u> that will help you to determine how healthy your back really is.

6. The <u>Opti-stretch Screening Exam</u> will allow you to identify the risk factors for recurrent back pain that you might have. The exam is both for adults and children.

7. The self-assessment Opti-stretch screening exam is reliable for most healthy individuals. However, a qualified instructor to administer the exam is even a better option. They can tell you with over a 90% probability whether you have a healthy back.

8. By decreasing or eliminating the <u>risk factors</u> for recurrent back pain through the Opti-stretch stretching exercises you can significantly improve your back problems.

9. It doesn't happen overnight and in many cases takes six months of hard work.

10. Don't let a bad back determine your activity level and lifestyle!

11. Take it from someone who has been there, the time and effort is definitely <u>worth it</u>.

Twelve – Opti-stretch Scientific Discoveries

■ ■ ■

1. Anatomic cause of Benign (Common) Back Pain.
   a. For over 300 years, it has been documented that a common form of low back pain is located over the sacroiliac joint. Many hundreds of researchers have attempted to identify the anatomical cause of this pain.
   b. Muscle complexes responsible for the majority of Benign Back Pain.
      i. Psoas Muscle Complex – for the lower back, sacroiliac area and hips.
      ii. Rhomboids – for the upper back [requires correction of (i)].
      iii. For the neck, the Trapezius has long been recognized. The new discovery is that correction of (i) and (ii) greatly facilitates rehabilitation.

2. Anatomical variability and physiologic complexity of the Psoas Muscle Complex.
   a. Several researchers have previously documented there are 3 different forms of the psoas muscle complex anatomy.
   b. Opti-stretch has discovered 2 other different forms of iliopsoas tendon length.
   c. This makes 18 different variants of the psoas muscle complex anatomy found in the general population.
      i. This correlates well with population statistics for back pain.
      ii. Helps explain the complexity of Benign Back Pain.
   d. Unless other accessory core muscles are first rehabilitated, the psoas muscle complex cannot be fully rehabilitated.

3. "Recurrent Back Strain Syndromes".
   a. "Psoas Short-Leg Low Back Strain".
      i. Functional leg shortening is nearly always seen.
      ii. Anatomic leg shortening is usually not a significant factor.
   b. "Rhomboid Upper Back Strain".
   c. "Trapezius Neck Strain".

4. "ACIM" (Asymptomatic Chronically Injured Muscle).
   a. The major cause of "recurrent back strain syndromes".
   b. Found only in certain core muscles.
   c. Can develop following acute injury if 100% healing does not occur.
   d. Accounts for the majority of asymmetry seen in body movement.
   e. Other causes of asymmetry include:
      i. Indirect muscle spasm due to Pathologic (Malignant) Back Pain.
      ii. Tendon and ligament shortening.

5. Determination of a healthy back or bad back (trick back).
   a. First need a Doctor's evaluation to check for Pathologic (Malignant) Back Pain.
   b. Potential for self-assessment and evaluation.

6. Scientific screening test to indicate whether you have a healthy back.
    a. Opti-stretch screening tests (Step 1 of the Opti-stretch Challenge).
        i. Beginning Program
        ii. Intermediate Program.
        iii. Advanced Program.
    b. Risk factor analysis of "recurrent back strain" (asymmetry greater than 1 inch).

7. Opti-stretch Therapeutic Technique (Step 2 of the Opti-stretch Challenge).
    a. "Stretch receptor lengthening".
        i. Incremental movement technique.
        ii. Incremental exhalation technique.
        iii. Forced exhalation.
    b. 2 to 6 months of work.
    c. Recognition of "secondary stretch receptors" past the age of 35.

8. Muscle Tone.
    a. Improved scientific definition.
    b. Accurate, yet simple measurement of the range of motion for core muscles.
    c. Objective measurement of the "first sensation of stretch".
    d. Four transition points for "stretch to pain transition" in healthy muscles.
    e. Aneroid manometer measurement.
    f. Potential for large scale standardization of healthy muscle tone for all of the various body types.

9. Maintenance (Step 3 of the Opti-stretch Challenge).
    a. Realistic and goal oriented stopping point.
    b. Time-efficient program.
    c. Cost effective.
    d. First aid for a life-time of healthy muscles.
    e. Activity level most precisely defines and best preserves a healthy back.

10. "Gold standard" for range of motion.
    a. Stretch receptor lengthening beyond this point appears to offer no significant improvement for rehabilitating a bad back.
    b. Not necessary in all body types.
    c. Screening test for genetic hyperflexibility.

11. Posture.
    a. Recognition of correctable factors (i.e., ACIMs).
    b. Improved awareness to help provide a life-time of optimum activity.

12. Involuntary (Instinctive) Stretching.
    a. Found in all non-aquatic mammals.
    b. Comparison to stretching exercises.
    c. Help in determining key stretching exercises.

Appendix A: Height-o-gram

■ ■ ■

This is simply a measurement of your height while standing on each foot separately. The height while standing on the right foot or the left foot may be the same or it may be several inches different.

The easiest way is to practice standing on one foot while balancing on the toes of the other foot. (See figure below. This is as viewed from the wall.) With a little practice, a smooth transition can be made from the left foot to the right.

A book works well to place on the head. The individual backs up until the bottom of the book is flush with the wall. This assures consistent distance from the wall and helps prevent rotation. A pencil is held by the individual or another person against a sheet of typing paper that has been taped to the wall.

From an equal weighted stance, the weight is transferred to the right leg and then to the left leg. This can be performed several times until a consistent tracing is obtained. Measure the difference between the right leg height and the left leg height. The shorter leg distance is recorded for your records. (See below)

Note that this distance may change several times during your life depending on the number of injuries and the extent of the injuries.

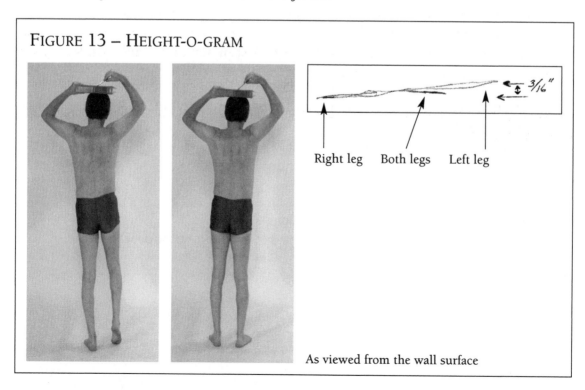

FIGURE 13 – HEIGHT-O-GRAM

Right leg   Both legs   Left leg

As viewed from the wall surface

APPENDIX B: INJECTIONS

■ ■ ■

Injections are not necessary for success in the Opti-stretch program. However, there may be a small percentage of the population who might be significantly helped by this technique.

In brief, this is a standard steroid injection with the proportions of ingredients described in prolotherapy injections. Injections are performed with a 2 cc amount of solution with a 23 gauge, 1 1/2 inch needle. The first injection is performed both directly through and no more than 2 centimeters anterior to the sacrolumbar ligament. The second is transabdominal but definitely not transperitoneal into iliacus muscle 4 cm below the anterior superior iliac spine. The third injection is into the iliopsoas muscle at the level of the anterior inferior iliac spine. Again, it is extremely important <u>not</u> to use a transperitoneal approach. The fourth is into the gluteus medius muscle and deep hip flexor at 2-cm superior to the most superior aspect of the greater trochanter. No more than 1-inch depth of needle insertion is utilized to insure no involvement with the hip joint.

Originally, a fifth area was attempted. This was into the iliopsoas muscle at the level of the groin. However, due to the lidocaine with epinephrine solution, the anterior cutaneous femoral nerve was frequently anesthetized. More importantly, the cutaneous anesthesia would resolve before the complete proprioception had returned to the knee. This made ambulation possible but any additional stress could tend to make the knee give away until the anesthetic effects of the injection had completely dissipated. The risk of a patient falling was not worth the benefit seen and only the four injections in the preceding paragraph were used.

At some point in time this injection technique may deserve some formal study and investigational trials.

Appendix C: Opti-stretch Intermediate Program

Example Values – Figure 14

■ ■ ■

Height-o-gram at Screening R _1 in, lower_ L_____	Ht 5'11"	Weight 189	Screening test		2 Month Opti-stretch Intervals			
Height-o-gram after Opti-stretch R _3/16 in lower_ L_____	Ht 5'11 _"	Weight 175	T= Tight		Before Warm-up		After Warm-up	
			R	L	R	L	R	L
1. Kneeling Nose to Floor			T		T		=	
					=		=	
					=		=	
2. Sitting Nose to Knee – (Figure Four) ***			in 8	in 6	8	6	7	5
					6	6	0	0
3. Supine Nose to Knee			in 6	in 4				
					2	2	0	0
4. Sitting Knees to Floor – (Butterfly) ***			in 5	in 4				
					1	1	0	0
5. Sitting Knee to Cross Chest			in	in				
6. Kneeling wide Stance Pelvis to Floor			T					
7. Kneeling Elbows Back to Floor			in	in				
8. Prone Twisting Crawl			In 2	in 1				
							3	2
9. Sitting cheerleader – Elbow to Ankle			In 12	in 9				
							4	3

			R	L		R	L	R	L
10. Sitting cheerleader – Nose to Knee		in	In				18	16	
11. Sitting cheerleader – Hip to Cross Knee							Tight		
12. Kneeling Narrow Stance Pelvis to Floor – (Cobra)							T		
13. Rhomboid pull		T					Equal		
14. Finger Touch		In 4	In 2				0	0	
15. Chin to Shoulder		In 2	In 0						
16. Chin Backwards			T						
17. Ear to Shoulder		in	In **T**						
18. Straight Arm Ear to Shoulder									
19. Chin to Chest			In 1				Equal	0	
20. Ear to Axilla (Armpit)			T						

*** Accurate measurements are important only in exercises 2 and 4.

APPENDIX D: OPTI-STRETCH INTERMEDIATE PROGRAM

WORKSHEET – FIGURE 15

■ ■ ■

Height-o-gram at Screening R_____L_____	Ht	Weight	Screening test		2 Month Opti-stretch Intervals			
Height-o-gram after Opti-stretch R_____L_____	Ht	Weight	T= Tight		Before Warm-up		After Warm-up	
			R	L	R	L	R	L
1. Kneeling Nose to Floor								
2. Sitting Nose to Knee – (Figure Four) ***			in	in				
3. Supine Nose to Knee			in	in				
4. Sitting Knees to Floor – (Butterfly) ***			in	in				
5. Sitting Knee to Cross Chest			in	in				
6. Kneeling wide Stance Pelvis to Floor								
7. Kneeling Elbows Back to Floor			in	in				
8. Prone Twisting Crawl			in	in				
9. Sitting cheerleader – Elbow to Ankle			in	in				

		R	L	R	L	R	L
10. Sitting cheerleader – Nose to Knee		in	In				
11. Sitting cheerleader – Hip to Cross Knee							
12. Kneeling Narrow Stance Pelvis to Floor – (Cobra)							
13. Rhomboid pull							
14. Finger Touch		In	In				
15. Chin to Shoulder		In	In				
16. Chin Backwards							
17. Ear to Shoulder		in	In				
18. Straight Arm Ear to Shoulder							
19. Chin to Chest			In				
20. Ear to Axilla (Armpit)							

*** Accurate measurements are only important in exercises 2 and 4.

Appendix E: Opti-stretch Beginning Program

Worksheet – Figure 16

■ ■ ■

Height-o-gram at Screening R_____ L_____	Ht	Weight	Screening test	2 Month Opti-stretch Intervals			
Height-o-gram after Opti-stretch R_____ L_____	Ht	Weight	T= Tight	Before Warm-up		After Warm-up	
			R	L	R	L	R	L
1. Kneeling Chest to Knee								
2. Supine Knee to Chest			in	in				
3. Supine Knee to Chest with Nose to Knee			in	in				
4. Supine Hip Hike			in	in				
5. Supine Knee to cross Chest			in	in				
6. Supine Straight Knee to Nose								
7. Sitting Knees to Floor			in	in				
8. Supine Both Knees to Chest			in	in				

APPENDIX F: DAILY ROUTINE USING THE OPTI-STRETCH SET

■ ■ ■

TABLE 4		
Phase	**"Say Aloud"**	**Description**
Start	Ready	Comfortably get into the general exercise starting position. Note, there should be no sensation of stretch on any of the muscles.
Detection	Check Check Check And Stretch Stretch Stretch And	At 1-2 second intervals, determine where the "first sensation of stretch" is for you. This is the onset of mild discomfort of stretch. Breathe in. Slowly and cautiously proceed to a second sensation of stretch in the muscles. This is often the beginning of moderate discomfort of stretch and is generally a safe range that you can work in. Return to the Ready position while taking in a breath.
Warm-up	Relax – 5 4 3 2 1 And Relax – 5 4 3 2 1 And	First stretch into mild discomfort intensity. Partially exhale at number increments. With improved muscle tone a slightly increased amount of range of motion can be accomplished without increasing the sensation of mild discomfort intensity. This is accomplished primarily by conscious relaxation of the muscles. Relax the stretch ½ inch while taking in a breath. Repeat as above. Inhale while relaxing the stretch 1-2 inches or more until comfortable. Repeat a third time.
Opti-stretch Subset 1 Opti-stretch Subset 2 Opti-stretch Subset 3	1 2 3 And 1 2 3 And 1 2 3 And* forced exhalation	While saying each number, exhale approximately ⅓ of the lung volume over a period of 1 second. Increase the stretch ¼ inch. (Do not exceed the predetermined level of stretch of mild, moderate or greater.) Inhale over 2 seconds while relaxing the stretch ½ inch. (If this level of stretch intensity is moderately uncomfortable, relax the stretch completely and start the subset again.) Repeat as Subset 1 and 2, except during <u>And*-ex</u>. Take in only a very small breath (or even better, none at all). Then exhale totally by contracting the chest wall muscles to force out the residual volume. <u>**Remember**</u> to never exceed 1 inch of additional range of motion. Then slowly relax the stretch completely. Repeat 3 times.

Table 4 (continued)

1. After performing an Opti-stretch set, rest the muscles at least 1 minute. Either perform the same exercise on the opposite side of the body or perform a similar exercise in the same general position (i.e., prone, kneeling or sitting).

2. Then repeat the set. If the muscles appear to be warmed up (which usually takes a week or two of practice to determine), proceed to your predetermined increased level of intensity. After two weeks of practice, this is usually to the moderate level. Following 2 months of practice this can maximally proceed to the moderately severe intensity level.

3. The intensity level is repeated usually twice on each side. Once a full one or two inches of increased range of motion has been achieved, (which usually takes 2 months), a total of three sets can be performed on the tighter side and two sets on the side that has the increased range of motion in order to narrow the asymmetry.

4. The maximum number of sets at the mild intensity level is determined by the amount of time one has to exercise a day. However, due to fatigue of the muscles, only 3 sets should be performed at any moderate intensity level or higher for a given exercise stretching session. In my experience, after this number of maximum predetermined sets, little is gained, time efficiency is decreased and the risk of injury increases significantly. "More is not always better."

5. The number of exercise sessions per day can be as frequent as one every hour. This type of time commitment is usually unrealistic for the average individual. However, performing two or three exercise sessions per day on the weekends can significantly accelerate your progress. Exercise sessions can be broken down into abbreviated sessions of 2-4 exercises. Remember, with the warm up built into each exercise, if you have an extra 5 minutes of time a couple of exercises can be performed. (This is one type of exercise session that you don't feel like you have to hit the showers upon completing.)

6. For the first 2-8 weeks, you need to be gentle and careful with your muscles. At the end of each exercise session you should feel as if you just had a relaxing deep muscle massage. (For many this can be a great and effective long-term level of exercise. For others, the intensity level has to be increased to achieve the results they desire. Still, the knowledge of performing the exercises to the level of a relaxing deep muscle massage is valuable for cool downs after sports, giving the muscles a little rest after days of intense workout or just relieving a little stress of the day. (This can be particularly beneficial for those who have trouble falling asleep.)

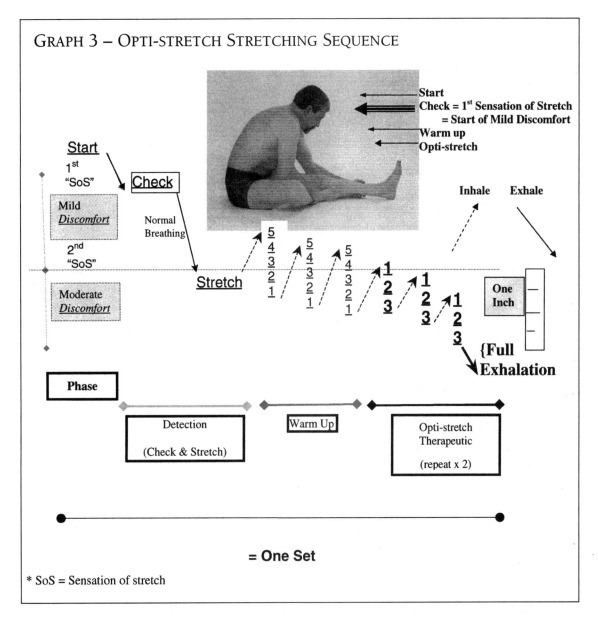

GRAPH 3 – OPTI-STRETCH STRETCHING SEQUENCE

Start
Check = 1ˢᵗ Sensation of Stretch
= Start of Mild Discomfort
Warm up
Opti-stretch

Start
1ˢᵗ "SoS"

Mild *Discomfort*

2ⁿᵈ "SoS"

Moderate *Discomfort*

Check

Normal Breathing

Stretch

Inhale   Exhale

5 4 3 2 1   5 4 3 2 1   5 4 3 2 1

1 2 3   1 2 3   1 2 3   1 2 3

One Inch

{Full Exhalation

Phase

| Detection (Check & Stretch) | Warm Up | Opti-stretch Therapeutic (repeat x 2) |

= **One Set**

* SoS = Sensation of stretch

Note: One Intermediate Set = Detection Phase, Warm Up Phase and <u>three</u> Opti-stretch Therapeutic Phases

Index

■ ■ ■